# KEEPING FIT ALL THE WAY

## How to Obtain and Maintain Health, Strength and Efficiency

## WALTER CAMP

# Keeping Fit All the Way

## Walter Camp

© 1st World Library – Literary Society, 2004
PO Box 2211
Fairfield, IA 52556
www.1stworldlibrary.org
First Edition

LCCN: 2005901392

Softcover ISBN: 1-4218-1194-4
Hardcover ISBN: 1-4218-1094-8
eBook ISBN: 1-4218-1294-0

Purchase *"Keeping Fit All the Way"*
as a traditional bound book at:
www.1stWorldLibrary.org/purchase.asp?ISBN=1-4218-1194-4

1st World Library Literary Society is a nonprofit
organization dedicated to promoting literacy by:

- Creating a free internet library accessible from any computer worldwide.
- Hosting writing competitions and offering book publishing scholarships.

***Keeping Fit All the Way***
*contributed by Tim, Ed & Rodney*
*in support of*
*1st World Library Literary Society*

# TABLE OF CONTENTS

# INTRODUCTION

The number of men who "keep fit" in this country has been surprisingly few, while the number of those who have made good resolutions about keeping fit is astonishingly large. Reflection upon this fact has convinced the writer that the reason for this state of affairs lies partly in our inability to visualize the conditions and our failure to impress upon all men the necessity of physical exercise. Still more, however, does it rest upon our failure to make a scientific study of reducing all the variety of proposals to some standard of exceeding simplicity. Present systems have not produced results, no matter what the reason. Hence this book with its review of the situation and its final practical conclusions.

# AN AMERICAN CITIZEN'S CREED

I believe that a nation should be made up of people who individually possess clean, strong bodies and pure minds; who have respect for their own rights and the rights of others and possess the courage and strength to redress wrongs; and, finally, in whom self-consciousness is sufficiently powerful to preserve these qualities. I believe in education, patriotism, justice, and loyalty. I believe in civil and religious liberty and in freedom of thought and speech. I believe in chivalry that protects the weak and preserves veneration and love for parents, and in the physical strength that makes that chivalry effective. I believe in that clear thinking and straight speaking which conquers envy, slander, and fear. I believe in the trilogy of faith, hope, and charity, and in the dignity of labor; finally, I believe that through these and education true democracy may come to the world.

WALTER CAMP

# PART I

# KEEPING FIT ALL THE WAY

# CHAPTER I

It has long been a startling fact regarding Americans that so soon as their school-days were over they largely abandoned athletics; until, in middle life, finding that they had been controverting the laws of nature, they took up golf or some other form of physical exercise.

The result of such a custom has been to lower the physical tone of the race. Golf is a fine form of exercise, but in an exceedingly mild way. No one claims that it will build up atrophied muscles nor, played in the ordinary way, that it will induce deep breathing; nor, except in warm weather, that it will produce any large amount of skin action. Hence it is easy to imagine the condition of the man who at the end of his 'teens gave up athletics, and then did nothing of a physically exacting nature until he took up golf. Now if in addition to his pastime and relaxation he will do something in the way of setting-up exercises to open up his chest and make his carriage erect, thus enabling his heart and lungs to have a better chance, he will more than double the advantages coming from his golf. He will then walk more briskly and will gain very much in physical condition.

## NATURE A HARD MISTRESS

One thing that our middle-aged men, and in fact many of

us who have not yet reached that way mark, have entirely forgotten is that Nature is very chary of her favors. Our primal mother is just and kind, but she has little use for the man who neglects her laws. When a man earns his bread by the sweat of his brow she maintains him in good physical condition. When he rides in a motor-car instead of walking she atrophies the muscles of his legs, hangs a weight of fat around his middle, and labels him "out of the running." If he persists in eating and not physically exerting himself, she finally concludes that he is cumbering the earth, and she takes him off with Bright's or diabetes. It does not do him any good to tell her that he was too busy to walk and so had to ride, or that he had no time for exercising; she simply pushes him off to make way for a better man.

## THE VICIOUS CIRCLE

Nature has given man two ways (outside of the action of the bowels) of getting rid of impurities, one by means of the skin and the other by means of the kidneys. It is like a motor-car with two cylinders. If one stops the other will run on for a time, but its wear is increased. When a man stops exercising and ceases to carry off by means of his skin some of these impurities, he throws an additional load on his kidneys. When a man goes without exercise and begins to accumulate fat, that fat gradually deposits itself and not alone about the waist; it invades the muscular tissue all over his body even to his heart. As this accumulation grows there come with it a muscular slackness and a disinclination to exercise. The man is carrying greater weight and with less muscular strength to do it. No wonder that when he tries to exercise he gets tired. He is out of condition. Hence he begins to revolve in a vicious circle. He knows that he needs exercise to help take off the fat, but exercise tires him so much, on account of the fat, that he becomes exhausted; usually he gives it up and lets himself drift again. As his abdomen becomes more pendulous his legs grow less active. As his energy wanes his carriage becomes more slack. He shambles along as best he can, if he is positively obliged to walk. His feet trouble him. Altogether he is only comfortable when riding. When he has reached this state the insurance companies regard him as a poor risk, and instead of enjoying the allotted threescore and ten years of real life he falls short by a decade; and even then the last ten years are but "labor and sorrow."


## AS THE YEARS GO ON

The first thing that a man begins to lose through the inroads of age is his resistive power. He may seem in perfect health so long as there is no special change of conditions, but when he is placed in a position where he needs his resistive forces to throw off disease, he finds that he cannot command them.

Still another change is continually taking place; as the man goes on in life, little by little the control of his muscles leaves him. Instead of running about as does the youth, recklessly and with never a thought of being tired, he begins to favor himself by walking in the easiest possible way, until soon he is balancing on one foot and then tilting forward on the other, making no muscular effort and preferring the motor-car or the trolley whenever it is at hand. As an inevitable result, some of the muscles atrophy, and even those that do not deteriorate speedily discover that they have no master, and they act when and how they please.

The man who is continually giving orders to subordinates and having other men do things for him, soon finds that he is unable to accomplish things for himself; then, if he is thrown on his own resources, he is helpless. Take a group of men, executives, who for a dozen years have been ordering other men about instead of obeying orders, and you will find that for the most part these captains of industry have lost 50 per cent. of their muscular control. On the other hand, the man who is taking orders retains command over all his muscles, for he is daily and hourly training them to instant obedience. A group of privates will snap into "attention" at the word of command with splendid muscular control; the same number of officers would find great difficulty in doing this. Now as the man loses muscular control he loses poise and carriage. His head rolls about in a slack way on his neck, and has a tendency to drop forward; the muscles of the neck and the upper part of the back grow soft from lack of use and control and he begins to become round-shouldered; his chest falls in as the shoulders come forward and the chest cavity is reduced. This means a gradual cramping of lungs, heart, and stomach.

By way of compensation he lets out a hole or two in his belt and starts in to carry more weight there. In other words, he exchanges muscle for fat, and as the fat increases he has less and less muscular strength to carry it. It is as though in a motor-car one added hundreds of pounds of weight to the body and reduced the horse-power of the engine. Pretty soon the man becomes so heavy around the waist that he notices his discomfort, and it produces exhaustion; now he becomes more and more averse to exercise, and the facia, or fat, having the better of the battle, begins to penetrate even the fiber of the muscles.

## THE REMEDY

The heart is a muscle, like all the others in the body, and fat may accumulate there. When this condition comes about the man is perforce obliged to be careful, for the heart muscle has lost its strength. As stated, the situation becomes a vicious circle: as the man adds fat he becomes more and more averse to exercise, and the less he exercises the fatter he gets. And yet all this can be prevented; nor is it necessary to take up any violent system of training, or to engage in tremendous gymnastic exercise. If the patient is willing to take reasonable physical training along scientific lines, a few hours a week will keep him in respectable shape, so that he may preserve not only his figure, but also his activity.

It should be remembered that all the members of the body partake of the slackness that is apparent externally. Thus organs that should be active in changing fat into energy lose their tone, and with that goes their ability to carry on their proper functions. The best work of the man himself is co-ordinated with the proper performance of the bodily activities. Growth and strength depend upon and react upon the tissues, and while this process is less active as age comes on, it can be stimulated to the great advantage of both mind and body.

## WHAT WORRY DOES

Every man who has reached a high place in his community or who has become a leader of note knows that executive work has a tremendous effect upon the nerves and body. If the man becomes run-down the smallest decision gives him difficulty; it seems weighted with enormous possibilities of disaster. A problem, which under normal conditions he would turn over with equanimity to his assistant, takes on, in his nervous state, a seriousness that leads to hours of worry. And yet if he goes away on a vacation he returns to find that nine-tenths of these troublesome things have been well taken care of during his absence. Moreover, now that he has come back in a state of physical health and with nerves that are normal, he sees that these awful problems were simply exaggerated in his own mind by his overwrought physical condition.

Few people realize the effect of worry upon the digestion.

An experiment was once tried upon a cat, which was fed a dish of milk, stroked until it purred, and played with for half an hour. The animal was then killed and the stomach examined; the milk was perfectly digested. Another cat was taken and given a similar saucer of milk; then its fur was rubbed the wrong way and it was teased and annoyed as much as possible for half an hour. Upon examining the stomach of the second cat it was found that not a step in the process of digestion had taken place.

## AMERICANITIS

It is wise to study the condition that we might almost call "Americanitis." The American youth, as shown in the Olympic games, is not only a match in speed, strength, and stamina for the youth of other nations, but when it comes to the individual specialist even then the American-trained boy is his superior. We smash records regularly. We have been doing this for a decade with hardly a break. Even those who criticize our tendency to develop individuals are obliged to admit that this continual advance in athletic prowess fosters the spirit of emulation among the masses. Moreover, we are improving in the way of distributing our efforts, and more and more men in schools and colleges come out for physical training and development. We have not by any means perfected the system, but it is on the way. Supplementing this general athletic development comes now the introduction into the curriculum of military drill.

Finally compulsory military education or at least the compulsory physical part of it, throughout the country will set up the youth of the coming race in a way hitherto unthought of. It is safe to say that the next decade will see our youth, and men up to the age of forty, in far better physical condition than is the case to-day.

## THE PRICE OF SUCCESS

The men of this country, with their forcefulness and their ambition, their stern desire to succeed quickly and to work furiously if necessary to obtain that success, are apt to forget that Nature meant man to earn his bread by the sweat of his brow; and that just so far as he departs from this primal method of supporting himself and his family he must pay toll. Almost before he realizes it the American youth is a staid man of business. Only yesterday he was a boy at play, and to-day he finds himself known by his first name or nickname only to a few old classmates whom he sees at his college reunions. He is Judge This or Honorable That. He has had no time to realize that somewhere he has lost fifteen or twenty years in this wild rush for fortune and fame.

Now in some hour of enforced reflection during a temporary illness he begins to count the cost, to think how little he has in common with that growing boy of his. But still he does no more than wish that he might have more time for play and could see his way to longer and less interrupted vacations. Perhaps on his next period of relaxation he plunges into an orgy of physical exercise - plays to the point of exhaustion - enjoys it, too, and sleeps like a log. Oh, this is the life once more!

When he returns to town he determines to take more time for exercise; he will keep up his tennis or golf. But once back at work, he must make up for lost time. He returns with an improved appetite and he indulges it. Soon his vacation benefits have worn off, together with his vacation tan. The muscles slacken again, the waistline increases. He feels a little remorse over the way he has broken his good resolutions, but of course he cannot neglect his business. Then, after a hard week, followed by some carelessness or exposure, he thinks that he has the grip or a cold. He is lucky if he stays at home and calls in his physician. He does not pick up. Now, for the first time, he hears from the doctor words that he has caught occasionally about men far older than himself - "blood pressure." But he he is under fifty! The doctor says he must go slower. Now begins a dreary round indeed! He has never learned to go slow! He is an old man at fifty. If lucky, he has made money. But what is the price? He has found precious little fun in those fifteen or twenty years since he was a boy. Of course he has had his high living, his motor, his late hours. His cigars have been good, but he has never enjoyed them so much as he did the old pipe at camp. His dinners and late suppers can't compare with the fish and bacon of the woods.

What a fool he has been!

Perhaps he has caught himself in time. If so he is in luck and Nature may partially forgive him and give him a chance to "come back." He is well scared and he means to be good. But the scare wears off, and then, too, "business" presses him on again. And finally, still well this side of sixty, perhaps, Nature taps him on the shoulder and says, "Stop!"

"But," he pleads, "I'll be good!"

"You are in the way," she replies, "and the sooner you make place for wiser men the better I shall have my work done."

But it is not alone the business world that is full of these untimely breakdowns. We lose many a man in the professional ranks with ten years of his best work before him, the man of ripened intellect, with his store of reading and experience - stopped oftentimes in the very midst of that masterpiece whose volumes would be read by future generations.

Executives whose value to corporations is increasing in a compound degree suddenly receive notice that the continually bent bow is cracking; almost immediately they lose their ambition and initiative, they become prematurely aged. These are indeed expensive losses!

And all this could be saved at an expenditure of a few paltry hours a week devoted to the repair of the physical man; given that and we may safely promise that he shall round out the full measure of his mental labors.

The men of this country are going the pace at a far more

reckless rate than that of any other nation. Philosophers like Prof. Irving Fisher are sounding the warning. Shall we heed it?

# CHAPTER II

When Dr. D.A. Sargent, of Harvard University, makes the charge that, "More than one-half of the male population between the ages of eighteen and forty-five years are unable to meet the health requirements of military service, and that, of the largest and strongest of our country folk pouring into our cities, barely one of their descendants ever attains to the third generation," it becomes a pretty serious charge. We are already familiar with the forgetfulness of physical condition by men over forty, but we had prided ourselves considerably over the belief that the majority of our youth would compare favorably with those of other countries. When one comes to sift the statement, he should remember that many disabilities for which the military examiners might reject a man are not so serious, after all, and that nothing has been said about the splendid physique of the large number of men who are accepted.

The writer visited recently many of the training-camps, both military and naval; and when he came away he was quite prepared to agree with those who praise the flower of the flock as being superior to that they have seen on the other side. The point is that Doctor Sargent is absolutely right in asserting that we ought not to have had so many rejections. It is time for us to realize that a man who is out of balance physically should be looked after. Moreover, men should not become out of balance.

The truth of the matter is that our mechanical devices have gone so far toward taking the place of manual labor that we only have one line of physical development - our athletic sports. If, therefore, these are not made broad enough and thorough enough and accessible enough, we are likely to have just what is happening now - namely, a slump when it comes to measuring up to the standard instituted by the military authorities.

Our young men do flock to the cities and city life means crowded conditions, lack of outdoor exercises, vitiated atmosphere, and a minimum of sunshine and of the other elements that go to perfecting and keeping up a robust and enduring physique.

## THE VALUE OF EXERCISE

Now exercise is the most important factor toward counteracting these unnatural conditions. Air, bathing, and diet aid, but we must have exercise in order to get the energetic contraction of the larger muscles of the body which goes so far toward regulating the physical tone. We must have what are called compensatory exercises, beginning as far down as the grammar-schools and continuing right through the universities and professional schools into general business and civic life. This war has opened our eyes; it should be a warning, and it ought to result in a far broader comprehension of what physical condition and physical education really mean. It is in this way only that we can meet the demands of modern civilization without an accompanying deterioration of the physical condition of our people. No one has set a finer example in this respect than President Wilson himself, who, realizing the enormous strain that was coming upon him, has systematically and conscientiously prepared for it. Early every morning, long before most Washingtonians are so much as turning over for their pre-getting-up nap, the President is out and off around the golf-course. Also Doctor Grayson has prepared a system of exercises for his use when outdoor work is impossible.

## PREPARING FOR EMERGENCIES

In the summer of 1917 several members of the Cabinet formed themselves into a club, with other prominent officials in Washington, and kept themselves fit throughout the season by consistent morning exercise, four days a week. So far so good, only we should have realized more than a year ago the strain that was coming upon our men and taken measures to meet it, as Germany did. Dr. William C. Woodward, who is chairman of the District Police Board in Washington, did not overstate the matter when he said that the draft officers were weary, that the strain had begun to threaten their efficiency, and that they were thoroughly undermining their bodies in the effort to accomplish their tremendous task. Every community has seen the same thing happen, and several of them can agree with Doctor Woodward that this has come close to being a really serious business calamity throughout the country. All these men should have been prepared by thirty or sixty days of physical training for this extra strain.

Again, the Equitable Life Assurance Society, in its September Bulletin, calls attention to the fact that, out of approximately 1,300,000 men who volunteered for the army and navy, only 448,859 were acceptable. Furthermore, the Equitable notes that these physical impairments not only will not correct themselves, but that they will get worse, and that a large percentage of our vast horde of physically sub-standard, low-priced men will drift into sickness and meet premature death because their power to resist disease is rapidly declining. The Equitable calls, on this convincing evidence, for a thorough and permanent system of health education in our schools, saying: "With all of our wealth and intelligence and scientific knowledge in the field of health conservation, we are allowing a large proportion of our children to pass out of the schools into adult life physically below par." The Equitable concludes with the remark: "Some day we will give all American school children thorough physical training and health education. Why not commence now?"


## FROM A FAMOUS PHYSICIAN'S NOTE-BOOK

Dr. S. Weir Mitchell says:

> All classes of men who use the brain severely, and who have also - and this is important - seasons of excessive anxiety or grave responsibility, are subject to the same form of disease; and this is why, I presume, that I, as well as others who are accustomed to encounter nervous disorders, have met with numerous instances of nervous exhaustion among merchants and manufacturers.

> My note-books seem to show that manufacturers and certain classes of railway officials are the most liable to suffer from neural exhaustion. Next to these come merchants in general, brokers, etc.; then, less freq-uently, clergymen; still less often, lawyers; and, more rarely, doctors; while distressing cases are apt to occur among the overschooled young of both sexes.

Here is a day's list:

Charles Page Bryan, former ambassador to Japan, died in Washington of heart failure at the age of sixty-one.

Judge Arthur E. Burr, Judge of Probate for Suffolk County, dropped dead in the court-house at the age of forty-eight.

Hiram Merrick Kirk, Municipal Court Justice, New York, died in the forty-seventh year of his age.

Lieut. William T. Gleason dropped dead in the railroad station, Salt Lake City, as he stepped from a railroad train, at the age of forty.

Indeed, it is not only the men of military age who drop off under this strain, but the very vital strong men behind the lines.

## THE ROAD TO EFFICIENCY

It is an extraordinary thing that the people in this country, many of them coming from the most vigorous ancestry, should be willing to compress all their athletic enthusiasm into a very small period of their school and college life, and then to forget to take any exercise (except vicariously) until warned, sometime after forty, that Nature will exact a price for such folly. It is certainly a puzzle to understand how men can willingly slip into fatness and flabbiness or nervous indigestion, forget entirely what a pleasure physical vigor is, fold their hands contentedly, with the statement that they haven't time for physical culture, and so, gradually, by way of the motor-car and the dinner-table, slide into physical decadence and a morbid condition of mind and body. And yet three or four hours a week, less than an hour a day, with the assistance of fresh air and water, and within a sixty-or ninety-day period, will start these people on the road to recovered health and vigor. All that is necessary is to get the proper action of the lungs, of the heart, and of the skin, and, finally, of the digestion; then the results will follow fast.

## A WINTER VACATION

The first time a good conservative New England business or professional man, who has worked hard all his life and who has attained a commanding position in the community, determines to break away and take a vacation in the winter - a thing he has heard about and sometimes wondered how other people could manage to do it - he meets with the surprise of his life. After boarding a train and traveling for twenty-four hours toward the South and sunshine, he begins to lose a little the feeling that he is playing "hookey" and is liable to be dragged home and birched. But he does wonder a little whether he won't have hard work in finding somebody to play with him. When, however, he disembarks from his train at his destination - we will say Pinehurst - he has already begun to realize, through noting the other bags of golf-clubs on the train, that possibly he will be able to get some partners. When he arrives at the hotel, although it is early breakfast-time, he is astounded at the number of people there, and he is inclined to think that he has happened upon an unusual week or that this is the one place in the South where golfers congregate.

By the time he has spent a day or two there and has

found that, in spite of the three courses open, it is wise to post his time the day before or he is likely to kick his heels around the first tee for a couple of hours before he can get away, and when he looks over the crowded dining-room at night - well, he comes to the conclusion that most of the school have deserted and are playing truant, too!

## THE GOSPEL OF FRESH AIR

A generation ago the people who preached the good gospel of fresh air were still viewed askance, although the new doctrine had begun to make some impression. The early settlers in this country lived an outdoor life perforce, and undoubtedly found all the excitement of a football game in fighting the Indians; consequently, they attained proper physical development. The descendants of these settlers still retained a good deal of the outdoor habit, but in the third generation the actual drift city-ward began. This meant the absence of incentives to outdoor exercise, so far as life and the pursuit of happiness were concerned. Hence, it became necessary to preach the gospel of fresh air.

"Oh, the joy with which the air is rife," sang Adams Lindsay Gordon, one of the early preachers of this doctrine, and to-day thousands and tens of thousands are appreciating the truth of the saying. Not alone the boy at school or college with his football, baseball, and rowing, but the middle-aged man with his golf and tennis, and the old man tramping through the woods with the rod and gun, as he used to do thirty years ago, and as he will do to the end - all these know what fresh air means. Sunshine, through the medium of golf, has come to the life of thousands of middle-aged wrecks formerly tied to an office chair. No one can estimate the number of lives, growing aged by confinement in close rooms, by lack of exercise, and by the want of cheerful interest in something beside the amassing of dollars and cents, that have been saved and rendered happy through the introduction of this grand sport whose courses now dot the country from Maine to California, from the top of Michigan to the end of Florida.

Twenty years ago in this country a man who came to his office in a golf suit would have been regarded as demented, to say the least. To-day the head of the house in many a large business refuses to permit anything to interfere with his Saturday on the links. And this means that he and all the officers in the departments under him, instead of viewing with concern the interest of the men in outdoor sports - their devotion to baseball and football, to tennis, golf, and track athletics - are glad and willing that the great outdoors should have a real place in their lives. It is good business policy.

Something must make up to the later generations for the loss of the open air and outdoor work which the exigentcies of the olden times demanded of our ancestors, and that something has come in the shape of physical exercise. But golf and long vacations are for the comparatively rich. They are makeshifts rendered possible only by circumstances.


## UNLEARNED LESSONS

If a man determined, because his horse or his dog showed exceptional intelligence, that he would endeavor to develop that intelligence by setting the animal at mental tasks, and so gave it only the exercise that would come from moving about the room, and no fresh air or sunshine, no road-work or hunting - well, we are all quite familiar with what the result would be.

If a parent had a child who showed unusual mental precocity and thereupon forced the brain of that child, with no outdoors, no fresh air, no sunshine, and even to late hours, we all recognize that such action would be criminal. Yet probably 50 per cent, of our best executives, in their efforts to aid in the present emergency, are doing just what we are ready to condemn in the hypothetical cases given above. Some of these men, while still able to whip up their will into going on from day to day with the same exhausting program, finally conclude that unless they take a vacation they are going to break down. The doctor tells them so and they know it. Whereupon they rush off for a week or ten days; some of them enter upon an orgy of exercise, others relax into a somnolent state of lying around and thanking their stars that they can rest at last. They certainly do feel better and do improve, but they come back to work merely to begin the same old vicious round. They have had their lesson, but they have not learned it.

# CHAPTER III

This is a young nation. It began with the great gods of Life, Liberty, and the Pursuit of Happiness. And it fought a good fight in the War of Independence for Freedom and Equality. Then came the lesser gods of material success. They broke the nation apart. But it survived. Since the Civil War we have grown rich and fat, flaccid and spineless. We are like a great, careless boy with a rich father; our crops and material resources symbolize the rich father who is able to pay for all his son's foolishness. And so the youth has never stopped to think. But underneath that careless exterior there are muscle and character. For what is the history of Youth? If the youth is to become a real man he cannot be curbed to the extent of forgetting courage in an excess of caution. And the rush of our youth to the service showed this.

## THE SPIRIT OF YOUTH

An Englishman once writing of the tendency of the elders to blot out all the fire of youth with restrictive legislation, said, "It is a fearful responsibility to be young, and none can bear it like their elders." How can a youth whose blood is warm within sit like his grandsire carved in alabaster? He cannot and he will not, and that is the salvation of the race. It is the old story of the stag in the herd. He will see no other usurp his rights until he is too old to have any.

Let me tell you something of the history of these attempts by the elders to curb the everlasting spirit of youth. At one time they would have eliminated all the sports. But we didn't let croquet become the national game! You ask what this nation of ours will become, and in reply I ask you what will you make of your boys?

Statisticians tell us that 90 per cent. of the men who go into business fail. Do you want your boy to fold his hands and say that because the chances are against him he will not try at all?

Are you going to let him get such a maximum of old man's caution that he reduces to a minimum the young man's courage?

Make him strong and well, just as you wish the nation to be strong and sound. There will always be plenty of middle-aged failures to preach caution.

Teach your boy fair play and may the best man win.

Teach him that the true sportsman "boasts little, crows gently when in luck, puts up, pays up, and shuts up when beaten"; that he should be strong in order to protect his country. A boy may over-emphasize his sports, but he will get over that. They tell us about the good old times when boys at college spent all their time in study and loved one another. There never were any such times. The town-and-gown riots took the place of sports, that's all.

## ECONOMIC LOSSES

We are all of us very much interested in the life of an automobile tire, and it seems to speak to us in terms we can readily understand. But only the particularly wise and successful men of our generation know and appreciate how valuable the life of a man is when expressed in those same terms of good hard dollars. Many manufacturers in the last two or three years have awakened to the fact that when, they put in a man and he stayed with them only two or three months, or even, in the case of executives, two or three years and then dropped out, either to go elsewhere or on account of ill health, it was a very distinct loss. In other words, they had put a certain investment into the man and that investment should have been growing more valuable to them all the time.

Germany's General Staff, previous to this war, was working overtime, just as our Cabinet and National Board of Defense are doing now - namely, till midnight and beyond. But the German General Staff was taken out into the Thiergarten in the morning for from one to two hours of exercise as a beginning of the day.

It therefore sifts itself down to this: If we had an ordnance officer who fired a gun, that was tested for but two hundred rounds without heating, five hundred times and thus cracked it, he would probably be discharged. If the superintendent in a factory doubled the number of hours he was running his automatic machinery, and instead of doubling the amount of oil actually cut it in half and thus ruined the machines, he would be regarded as a fool. Yet we are letting our men, high in executive positions, heads of departments in the government, and leaders of manufacturing, transportation, and commercial interests, do this very thing. Is it possible that we regard them as less valuable to us in this emergency than machines and guns, that we should burn them out for lack of lubricant and rest or physical conservation?

## WARNING EXAMPLES

A railroad president not long ago said that he had not the time to take exercise or rest, that his salary was fifty thousand dollars a year, and that his company had just given him a bonus of fifty thousand; hence he could not shirk his responsibilities. He paid the full measure and was buried in six months from the time of the warning. In one issue of the New York *Evening Post* the following deaths were noted:

President Hyde, formerly of Bowdoin, fifty-nine years of age. Capt. Volney Chase, of the Navy, fifty-six years of age. Capt. Campbell Babcock, fifty years old. Colonel Deshon, fifty-three years old.

Our Cabinet officers and executives and the members of the Council of National Defense are likely to forget, in the excess of their patriotism and loyalty, that there is one edict higher than that of the greatest government in the world. When Nature gives an order there is no appeal to a higher court, and the excuse that a man has not the time to obey, or is doing something that his country most urgently needs, has no weight in that court. When Nature touches a man on the shoulder and says, "Stop!" he stops. The penalty of frayed nerves, overworked brains, and underworked bodies is failure of body and mind. The premonitory symptoms are irritability, quarreling, depression, fierceness and inefficiency of effort, and finally complete breakdown. Three to four hours a week physical exercise under a scientifically tested plan and arrangement will keep these men fit. Is the price in this emergency too high to pay?

## PHYSICAL FITNESS A VITAL FACT

Up to the time when this world conflagration started, a man's physical fitness was merely a matter of individual interest. The general health of the community was important, but that fact was not sufficiently pressing to do much more than attract the attention of the health boards, and perhaps a few recently organized and semi-philanthropic bodies. But suddenly there flamed out a war in Europe, and at once the countries involved found that upon the physical fitness of the people would depend their lives and freedom. It was no longer an academic question. It became an immediate and vital fact.

In September of 1914 the writer placed the following suggestion on the top of his syndicate athletic article:

AMERICANS AWAKE!

Guard your shores and train your men,
Teach your growing youth to fight;
Make your plans ere once again
Ships of foes appear in sight.

Teach new arts until you hold
In your bounds all things you need.
Then you can't be bought or sold;
From commercial bonds be freed!

If Manhattan rich you'd save,
If your western Golden Gate -
Train a field force, rule the wave.
Every day you're tempting fate!

Build the ships and train to arms,
Make your millions fighting strength
That shall frighten war's alarms
Ere they reach a challenge length.

He was immediately assailed as a militarist, and yet, had we but taken those preparatory steps, millions of lives might have been saved.

# CHAPTER IV

And thus we approach one of the problems which this book is designed to solve. There are eight million men in this country between the ages of forty-five and sixty-four. Probably we may count upon another million from the men of sixty-four to seventy who would be "prospects," as the mining-men say. These men represent nine-tenths of the financial and executive strength of the United States.

## THE SENIOR SERVICE CORPS

When I started the experiment of the Senior Service Corps at New Haven, in the spring of 1917, all my men were over forty-five, and several of them had passed the seventy mark; yet all found increased health and efficiency from the prescribed regime. There was a distinct gain, not only in health, but in spirits and in temper. Nerves that had been at high tension relaxed to normal. Effort that had seemed exhaustive became pleasurable. The ordinary problems of business or finance, once so apt to be vexatious, lost their power to produce worry. In fact, these men had renewed their youth; they had altered the horizon-line of advancing age, across which only clouds of doubt and appre-hension could be seen, to that of youth, radiant with the sunshine of hope and the promise of accomplishment.

This war has started some new thoughts and has given emphasis to others that may not be new but which have never been forced home. One of these is the value of physical efficiency. A social scientist said some twenty years ago that the "greatest nation of the future would be the one which could send the most men to the top of the Matterhorn." Nations now realize that in such a time as this all men up to forty may be required for the firing-line; and this means that all the men from forty to seventy must be rendered especially efficient and physically fit in order to stand back of the fighting forces as a dependable reserve - money, power, and brains.


THE BASIC IDEA

This was the idea of the development of the Senior Service Corps - to take men who are over military age and make them physically fit for whatever strain may come. It has resulted in not only making them physically fit, but in practically renewing their youth. The experimental (New Haven) company of a hundred, varying in age from forty-five to over seventy, in weight from 114 to 265 pounds, and in height from 5 ft. 4 in. to 6 ft. 4 in., after just completing ninety days' training, marched at the dedication of the Artillery Armory over four and one-half hours without physical discomfort.

Now, war or no war, the man of over military age would like to be fit, would like to feel that glow of youth which comes even to the man of fifty when he is physically in condition.

Nine-tenths of the men over forty-five can accomplish this, and they can do it by the expenditure of only three or four hours a week if they will follow with absolute care the rules demonstrated by a scientific experiment upon a company of one hundred men over a period of ninety days. This company of New Haven professional and business men included the president of the Chamber of Commerce, the editor of the largest evening newspaper, the dean of Yale University, the director of the gymnasium, the president of Sargent & Company, the owner of the Poli Theater Circuit, the ex-mayor of the city, two judges, the treasurer of the savings-bank, the registrar of Yale University, four professors, three doctors, and many leading corporation officials.

At the end of this period these men were not only able to march for over four hours without discomfort, but without losing a man. Moreover, they all gained in spirits, recovered their erect carriage, and found themselves enjoying their tasks.


COMMUNITY PHYSICAL DEVELOPMENT

The plan developed by the National Security League, under its committee on physical reserve, of assuring physical fitness for the nation, is capable of endless possibilities in application and development.

The plan treats each as a separate unit and allows it to adapt the physical-fitness scheme to local conditions, favoring the appointment of neighborhood groups for instruction in physical drill and the "Daily Dozen Set-up," assuring such conditions and applications of diet and hygiene as are particularly demanded by the individual community's conditions and demands.

Every individual detail and local development is left to

the committee which each mayor or town or borough official appoints, on invitation of the league.

The ideal toward which every community is working is the establishment, as an integral part of it, of a local fitness plant. This includes first, playgrounds laid out for all recreational sports, in their season. The ideal playground system will have enough room in walks and landscape-gardening for park development - sufficient to meet the community's maximum needs.

Community physical-fitness centers are growing up in which an adjacent lake or river provides facilities for rowing, canoeing, and recreational enjoyment through breathing the fresh air, while taking regular physical, conditioning exercises.

Such an ideal community plant has proven by no means a vision incapable of realization. To-day men and women realize painfully the need for one in their home community and are prevented from the fulfilment of their dream by only two obstacles - lack of funds and adequate organization of the plan.

This work and these centers offer the greatest possibilities in the Americanization scheme, perfection of which is a paramount duty for this country.

Not only do such plants transpose the astonishingly large percentage of the physically unfit of our foreign and domestic population and reclaim those whose physical imperfections have either become evident through the draft, or which are not known, but it affords the surest possible means of interesting this large element of our population in American institutions, of attracting them to the soundest and most beautiful features of American life, and of convincing them of their comradeship in the strength and sinew of American manhood; in short, of building the foundations of democracy on a base as stable as the eternal granite hills.


## AN OUTLINE OF THE SYSTEM

The Senior Service program starts with setting-up exercises which open the chest, gently stimulate the heart, and start the blood coursing through the system, and follows with progressive walking, a little hill-climbing, and, later in the development, with some weight-carrying exercises. The system renews the resistive force of the body, tones up the muscles, opens the chest cavity so that the heart and lungs have more room and the breath is deeper and better, gives general exercise to the various muscles which have become more or less atrophied from disuse, and brings about a marked improvement in the mental outlook and in the animal spirits.

The system is a combination of setting-up exercises with outdoor work, all carefully and precisely laid out after twenty years of experience in conditioning men. It should be followed absolutely, not partially or occasionnally. It is far from severe. Its strength lies in the cumulative effect rather than in any special effort at any one time.

It should be said that a mental effort is requisite in this course as well as the physical one. The correlation between mind and muscle must be re-established. The man must become master of his body once more and retain that mastery. Certain suggestions are also given specifically as to living - none of them irksome, but quite essential if the full result of the work is to be attained.

This was the first experiment of its kind, and hence it has proven of especial interest. There are plenty of cases of individuals taking up exercise in one form or another and benefiting somewhat by it; but when twenty to one hundred men in a group have engaged in this Senior Service work, the result has proven remarkable in every instance. The question seems to be simply this: If you are over military age and wish to renew your youth, and are willing to pay the price by devoting some three or four hours a week to a scientifically tested system, and can secure a score of other men to do it with you, you can be absolutely assured of success. Well, isn't it worth it?

## INDIVIDUAL AND GROUP ACTION

Thousands of men are beginning to realize what all this means. My mail for the last six months has been full of the inquiry. Men of forty are rapidly awakening and are eager to devote these few hours to the task of keeping fit, and so increasing their efficiency. At the same time they are preventing these horrible and untimely punishments at the hand of Mother Nature.

Now there are two methods by which a man may still be young at sixty. One is an exceedingly hard route for most men to travel - namely, the individual practice of this scientifically tested formula and patient persistence in it. The other is by group action. The latter is far easier and its results are doubly effective. However, as in some cases group action may be impossible, this book furnishes the data for individual practice as well.

All the exercises described are possible for the individual as well as for the group. Should a man determine to follow them out alone, he must make up his mind that there shall be no interference with his carrying out his program with regularity and exactness. He must not for a moment believe that he can miss the exercises one day and then make up for the lapse by doubling them the next day. He must always follow the setting-up exercises with his walk and not do the setting-up in the morning and then wait till afternoon for his walk. It is the combination that produces the most effective results.

In a group the leader constantly cautions the men as to carelessness or slackness. The individual having no leader must always keep his mind fixed upon the exact way in which his exercises should be performed. When he puts his hands behind his head in "Neck Firm" or "Head" he must keep his elbows back and his head up, while the chest should be arched. When he bends forward in the prone position he must not allow his head to droop. When he raises his knees in alternate motions he must bring his knees well up. When he does the exercise of leaning up against the wall, by means of the extended arm and hand, he must keep the distance far enough from the wall to bring about a certain amount of real effort by the hand, arm, and shoulder. And so it goes. It is for this reason that all the exercises are so carefully described and the method and manner of walking, marching, or "hiking" receive so much attention.

## WORK AND HYGIENE

In a book recently published by one of the highest

authorities on hygiene in the country, the following statements are made, statements which would prove of especial interest to those of us who have had the pleasure of being members of that "exclusive official Washington club," or of the Senior Service:

The problem of the mental worker is to get sufficient physical exercise to keep the mind and body at its maximum efficiency. This problem gets more and more acute as he gets older. The amount of work necessary to keep the man of sedentary habits in good condition is about 100 to 150 foot-tons. Five hundred foot-tons is the amount of work a soldier would perform by marching twenty miles at three miles an hour on a level road.

It is a fallacy to think that sufficient exercise can be taken once a week. In order to be efficient exercise must be regular and at relatively short intervals. All exercise should tend toward using all of the muscles of the body. In fatigue a person has lost control over his muscles. The process of getting into condition, therefore, is directed more toward strengthening the nervous system in its control work over the muscles rather than in increasing sheer muscular strength.

Pure creative mental work, although requiring no output of physical energy, is perhaps the most productive of fatigue. The brain gets more blood during physical activity and waste products are much better removed. The effects of exercise are particularly apparent in the lungs. More fresh air is brought to the lungs and the waste products are driven off.

An attainable minimum for the average adult person

might well consist of taking simple exercises in his room, and to get out of doors once a day and walk rapidly for at least half an hour. In addition, it is desirable for any one up to fifty years of age to take some kind of moderately violent exercise at least once a week. This should be sufficiently strenuous to induce perspiration. This is important for several reasons. In the first place, there is an old saying, which happens to be true, "Never let your blood-vessels get stiff." In addition we should call on the tremendous reserve which Nature gives to us, at least once in a while.

## WATER, WALKING, AND FOOD

Water plays a very important part in the life of man, for without it a person can live for only a short time. Its importance is shown by experimental fasts lasting for thirty days where only water was taken, and when we consider that the body is composed of from 60 to 70 per cent, of water and that the amount which it throws off as waste has to be replaced through nutrition, we realize the value of water to life. The average person, therefore, should take from two to four quarts of water a day.

At middle age it is natural for most people to put on weight, unless they are especially active in their daily life. For, having acquired a habit of consuming a certain amount of food, it is absolutely essential to exercise and thereby offset the tendency of this food to make fat and increase the weight. Walking can be enjoyed by everybody, and a four-or five-mile "hike" daily makes your credit at the bank of health mount up steadily. We should all learn that when we rob the trolley company of a nickel by walking we add a dime to our deposit of health.

Food, of course, is one of the main factors in one's general health, and we hear on all sides the opinions of people as to the causes of indigestion and the general ailments connected with eating. One thing is certain, however, and that is that pleasure has a favorable effect on the digestion. Pleasant company at a meal, the dainty serving of the viands, and the attractiveness of the food combinations pave the way to a satisfactory repast, eaten with enjoyment and completely assimilated.

## A MODEL DIETARY

Because diet is a real aid to physical well-being, the following table is offered as a rough suggestion for a typical dietary for a man leading a more or less sedentary life. But it will never replace exercise.

| BREAKFAST | Approximate Calories |
|---|---|
| Orange or grapefruit | 100 |
| Two eggs | 166 |
| Two Vienna rolls | 258 |
| Butter | 119 |
| Coffee with milk and sugar | 100 |
| Total | 743 |

| LUNCHEON | Approximate Calories |
|---|---|
| Twelve soda crackers | 300 |
| One pint milk | 325 |
| Total | 625 |

| DINNER | Approximate Calories |
|---|---|
| Soup (consomme) | 14 |
| Roast beef | 357 |
| Potato | 145 |
| String beans or peas | 13 |
| Bread | 100 |
| Butter | 119 |
| Apple pie | 352 |
| Glass of milk | 157 |
| | ---- |
| Total | 1257 |

Many people have adopted a so-called vegetarian diet, believing that it is better for the health than eating meat. Undoubtedly food from the vegetable kingdom is a great benefit to the human system, but strict vegetarianism is not recommended by our medical men. Nature apparently intended us to be omnivorous, and, in addition, vegetarianism may run too close to the dangers of carbohydrate excess. As man progresses after middle life he can unquestionably diminish materially the amount of meat in his diet.

In recent years there has been a revival of the theory of prolonged mastication of a limited amount of food. This theory is sound in so far as it tends to overcome the bolting of food and over-eating, but there is a belief among our practitioners that there is little basis in science or experience for the extremes of this character.


## HYGIENIC CURE-ALLS

Among recent fads is the so-called buttermilk or sour milk diet as advocated by Metchnikoff. The original theory was interesting and was, in part, that the bacteria derived from soured milk would drive out of the intestinal canal all the harmful germs. Quite possibly there may be something in the theory, especially if large quantities of milk are taken with the lactic acid bacilli, but the beneficial effect of this change of bacteria is not convincingly of great consequence.

## FRESH AIR

It is now generally known that an abundant supply of moving, pure, fresh air is the proper and simple solution of the problem of the hygiene of the air.

Oxygen is the element of the air which sustains life. We inhale about seven pounds per day, two pounds of which are absorbed by the body. The air becomes dangerous, or infected, when the oxygen in the air is decreased to only 11 or 12 per cent., and when the oxygen reaches 7 per cent. death occurs from asphyxiation.

The human body requires about three thousand cubic feet per hour, and the great problem of ventilation is to give this amount of pure air, moving, and with the proper amount of moisture.

It is a common belief that with each breath we take we are filling our lungs with fresh air. This is not the case, for we never do get our lungs filled with fresh air. What really happens is that we ventilate a long tube which has no intercommunication whatever with the blood. Most of the time our lungs are filled with impure air, and we simply exchange a part of it for fresh air.

# THE VALUE OF DEEP BREATHING

Deep breathing is undoubtedly extremely beneficial. Most of us, due largely to the fact that Nature leaves a considerable margin of safety, are able to carry on our ordinary activities without the requisite ventilation of the lungs, especially if we do not exercise. This, however, is injurious to the lungs, for it allows the blood to stagnate in them. Exercise is Nature's method of compelling ventilation in the lung area. Deep breathing may be used as a substitute, but the other beneficial effects of exercise are lost.

The skin and the various glands connected with it form a complex organism, the functions of which play a very important part in the work which the body has to do. The skin aids the lungs in their work of respiration; and, like the lungs, it throws off water and carbon dioxide and absorbs oxygen. The respiratory work of the skin, however, is only a minute fraction of that which the lungs do.

The skin is a heat regulator, and in this, its most important work, it is aided by the two million or more sweat-glands which are distributed over almost the entire surface of the body. The skin and the sweat-glands work together to keep the blood at an even temperature, either by giving off heat or in preventing this process in case the outside air is too cool. The body temperature, as a rule, is higher than that of the outside air, so that heat is generally being given off by the skin. We are perspiring constantly, but usually to such a slight extent that the fact is hardly noticeable. The amount of heat which is thrown off at any time is proportional to the amount of the tissue burned up by muscular action.

# CHAPTER V

Health, strength, and efficiency! Surely every man in this great Republic of ours wants to be healthy, strong, and efficient, but how is he to obtain and maintain this threefold blessing? It has been stated that scientific physical exercise, preferably taken in group association, will accomplish it. Now to consider some of the practical details involved.

## THE ORGANIZATION

The organization may be composed of any number from sixteen to one hundred men, and about the smallest unit that should be undertaken is that of sixteen men. On the other hand, when the number gets above one hundred (or preferably ninety-six, in order that it may be divided into four companies of twenty-four each) it is better to start a second group under a separate leader.

The first thing to do in the organization is to enroll at least one physician, who becomes the surgeon of the company. His name, together with that of the secretary of the unit, should be filed with the Senior Service Corps, of New Haven, Connecticut, or with the National Security League, of New York City, in order that any additional information or directions may be forwarded promptly.

The division of labor in the work should be from ten to fifteen minutes of the setting-up exercises, and from forty-five to fifty minutes of the outdoor work. It has been found upon scientific test that this is the best division, and the outdoor work should follow the setting-up exercises immediately, since the men are then in condition to benefit from the fact that they have opened up their chest cavity and are taking in more fresh air and oxygen.

The best way to start a unit is to get ten or a dozen leaders together at dinner or luncheon and organize; then pick out other men who are of importance in the community and add them to the charter number.

The editors of the local papers are usually very glad to lend their powerful assistance toward the project.

It is not necessary to have the outdoor work partake of the nature of military drill, but a certain amount of this, added after the second or third week, lends interest and also produces excellent results in muscular control.

In order to understand the various prescribed movements and exercises the following explanations should be carefully studied, of course, in connection with the illustrative photographs.


TO THE LEADER

It is particularly necessary that the leader should thoroughly familiarize himself with the movements and positions, for many of the men will not take the trouble to study the manual by themselves, or they may be unable to spare time for anything but the actual drill. It is the leader's business to instruct, and the progress of his squad or company will be in direct proportion to his knowledge and capacity to inspire real interest in and enthusiasm for the work.

Each movement must be executed perfectly and exactly or the benefit therefrom will not be fully assured. Much depends upon the leader; a man should be selected who has the gift of leadership.

## GIVING THE COMMANDS

In giving the commands care should be taken to discriminate between the explanatory and executive parts of the order, making a decided pause between. For example, in "Forward March!" "Forward" is the explanatory or warning word; then, after a perceptible pause, the executive word "March!" should be given in a crisp, decisive tone of voice. The command "Attention!" is but one word, but it is the custom to divide it syllabically, thus, "Atten-shun!" All other commands taken from the military manuals have their proper warning and executive words; for example: "Count - Off!" "About - Face!" "Right - Face!" "Company - Halt!" "To the Rear - March!" "Double Time - March!" etc. The exceptions are the commands, "Rest!" "At Ease!" and "Fall Out!"

The orders for the exercise movements may be standardized by first giving the name of the movement, "Arms Cross," and then adding the words: "Ready - Cross!" to indicate the second or executive part of the command. For example: "Arms Cross. Ready - Cross!" the men taking the "cross" position at the last word. In this way the members of the squad are first warned as to just what they are expected to do; then, at the executive word, they all act together. The leader should see to it that the over-eager men do not anticipate the executive command.

The only purely military formation used in this manual is that of the squad. Nowadays, when military training is so universal, the meaning of the term is well known; there is sure to be some one in the company who can supply the necessary information about forming the squad and the simple movement of "Squads Right." To put it into untechnical language, it may be said that the squad consists of eight men, lined up four abreast in two ranks. The men should be arranged in order of height, the tallest being No. 1, front rank. No. 4 of the front rank acts as corporal of the squad.

"Squads Right" looks like a complicated maneuver when studied according to the diagrams in the manuals, but it is not particularly difficult in practice. Its use is to get the company out of the double line formation into a column of four men abreast, the usual marching formation. At the executive command, "March!" No. 1 front rank acts as the pivot, and makes a right-angled turn to the right, marking time in that position until the three other men in the front rank have executed a right-oblique movement and have come up on the new line. The rear-rank men follow suit, but Nos. 2 and 1 have to turn momentarily to the left in order to get behind the front-rank pivot men - to put it more simply, they follow No. 2 in single file.

It sounds confusing, but any old National Guardsman can explain the movement in very short order. So soon as "Squads Right" has been completed the whole column takes up the march without further word of command.

## STEPS AND MARCHINGS

All steps and marchings executed from a halt (except Right or Left Step) begin with the left foot.

The length of the full step in "Quick (or ordinary) time" is 30 inches, measured from heel to heel, and the cadence is at the rate of 120 steps to the minute.

The length of the full step in "Double Time" is 36 inches; the cadence is at the rate of 180 steps to the minute.

## FORWARD - MARCH!

At the warning command, "Forward!" shift the weight of the body to the right leg, left knee straight. At the command, "March!" move the left foot forward 30 inches from the right; continue with the right and so on. The arms swing freely.

## DOUBLE TIME - MARCH!

The arms are raised to a position horizontal with the waist-line, fingers clenched. The run is as natural as possible.

## TO THE REAR - MARCH!

At the command, "March!" given as, the right foot

strikes the ground, advance and plant the left foot, turn to the right-about on the balls of both feet, and immediately step off with the left foot.

## COMPANY - HALT!

At the command, "Halt!" given as either foot strikes the ground, plant the other foot as in marching; raise and place the first foot by the side of the other. If in "Double Time," drop the hands by the sides.

## MARK TIME - MARCH!

At the command, "March!" given as either foot strikes the ground, advance and plant the other foot; bring up the foot in the rear and continue the cadence by alternately raising each foot about two inches and planting it on line with the other.

Being at a halt, at the command, "March!" raise and plant the feet in position as prescribed above.

## CHANGE STEP - MARCH!

At the command, "March!" given as the right foot strikes the ground, advance and plant the left foot; plant the toe of the right foot near the heel of the left and step off with the left foot.

The change as the left foot strikes the ground is similarly executed.

## RIGHT - FACE!

Raise slightly the left heel and right toe; face to the right, turning on the right heel, assisted by a slight pressure on the ball of the left foot; place the left foot by the side of the right. "Left Face" is executed on the left heel in a corresponding manner.

## ABOUT - FACE!

Carry the toe of the right foot about half a foot-length to the rear and slightly to the left of the left heel (without changing the position of the left foot); face to the rear, turning to the right on the left heel and right toe; place the right heel by the side of the left. There is no left "About Face."

## COUNT - OFF!

At this command all except the right files (the two men forming the extreme right end of the company as drawn up in two lines) execute "Eyes Right"; then, beginning on the right, the men in each rank count one, two, three, four - one, two, three, four, etc. As each man calls off his squad number he turns head and eyes to the front.

## THE SETTING-UP EXERCISES

Attention!

This is the regular military position. Heels together, the feet at an angle of forty-five degrees; hands at the sides, thumbs along seam of the trousers; neck back, chin in, chest out. (See Fig. 1.)

The movement calls for prompt control of the muscles; in fact, the expression is often used of "snapping into attention," meaning that the man comes into this position quickly and easily and with a distinct click of the heels. In the "Daily Dozen" referred to later in this book, this position is called "Hands."

Arms Cross (Ready-Cross!)

This movement is taken from the position of "Attention" by raising the arms from the sides and turning the palms down; it may be varied by turning the palms up. Holding the arms in this position, at the same time turning the hands and keeping the neck straight and the chest arched, will develop all the muscles over the shoulder. (See Fig. 2.)

On the "Cross" position the arms should be straight out horizontally from the body, with the elbows locked. At the same time, resistance should be placed against the head and neck coming forward at all. These should be held in exactly the same position as at "Attention." The tendency is either to let the arms bend a little or to let them drop below the horizontal, or even to hold them slightly above the level.]

From this position "shoulder-grinding" may be practised. This is executed by keeping the arms extended, turning the whole arm in a circle in the shoulder socket, and forcing the shoulder-blades back and together as the arms go back. The circle made by the hands should be about twelve inches in diameter.

Arms Stretch (Ready-Stretch!)

In this exercise the arms are raised to a position straight up above the head, with the hands extended. The palms may be together or facing front. (See Fig. 3.)

Hips Firm!

(This order is given, "Hips-Firm!")

The hands are placed on the hips, with thumbs back and fingers forward. The chest should be arched, the shoulders and elbows kept well back, and the neck pushed hard against the collar. (See Fig. 4.)

Also the hips should be kept well back and the abdomen in. This gives the same poise as the "Attention" position, but it puts more work on the shoulder muscles and so gives greater opportunity for arching the chest. In the "Daily Dozen" this position is called simply, "Hips."

Neck Firm!

(This order is given, "Neck-Firm!")

Maintaining the same position as in "Hips Firm," the hands are quickly raised and put against the back of the head (the finger-tips slightly interlaced) just where it joins the neck, exerting some pressure; at the same time the head and neck are forced well back. (See Fig. 5.)

The elbows should not be allowed to come forward, but should be kept back and the chest should be arched. This gives extra work for the muscles of the neck, as well as for those of the arms and shoulders. In the "Daily Dozen" this is called simply, "Head." (See Fig. 6.)

## Arms Reach (Ready-Reach!)

While maintaining an erect position, the arms are stretched out forward parallel to each other, the shoulders being kept back and the chest not cramped. If the shoulders are allowed to come forward the exercise is valueless. (See Fig. 7.)

## Arms Bend (Ready-Bend!)

In this position the arms are bent at the elbows, with the hands partially clenched, and brought up about to the point of the shoulders. The shoulders are held back firmly and the neck is pressed against the collar, while the chest is arched (Fig. 8). From this position the following movements are made with the hands clenched: Arms Cross (Ready-Cross)![1]

A good exercise in rhythmic time may be developed by going through the following round of movements: "Arms Bend, Arms Cross, Arms Bend, Arms Stretch, Arms Bend, Arms Reach, Arms Bend, Arms Down."

## Body Prone (Ready-Bend!)

Assuming the position of "Neck Firm," press the hands against the back of the neck and bend body at the waist forward, at the same time keeping the head in line with the spinal column and the eyes up; then back again to the erect position. (See Fig. 6a, Chapter XI.)

This gives excellent exercise for the muscles of the neck, and, if performed slowly, some exercise for the back.

Assuming the same position of "Neck Firm," bend the body slightly at the waist. This exercise should not be carried to an extreme, especially in the case of men who have reached middle age. In the "Daily Dozen" this is called "Grasp."

## Balancing (Ready-Balance!)

Assume the position of "Attention," then, standing on the right foot and keeping the knees straight, advance the left foot forward about two feet from the ground. Hold this position while balancing on the right foot, then back to "Attention" again. (See Fig. 9.)

Make the same motion, standing on the left foot. Now standing on the right foot, advance the left foot and, instead of bringing it to the ground, swing it back and extend it at the same height to the rear, still balancing on the other foot. Hold this position for a moment. After some practice this movement can be executed by standing on one foot and putting the other leg first forward and then back for several times.

This exercise gives control over the muscles of the leg and balancing powers, and increases the ability to adjust the muscles so as to maintain the equilibrium.

## Stride Position (Ready-Stride!)

This position calls for the separation of the feet sideways

about a foot and a half apart (Fig. 10). Now assume the "Arms Cross" attitude, and then, turning the body at the hips, bring first the right hand down to touch the floor, at the same time bending the right knee and keeping the left knee straight. Come back to the regular position again.

Now bend the left knee, put down the left hand and touch the ground, turning the body at the hips. (See Fig. 11.)

In both of these movements keep the other arm extended backward. This produces a graceful exercise which is excellent work for the muscles of the body and shoulders. In the "Daily Dozen" this is called "The Weave."

Assuming the "Stride Position," advance the right foot about a foot; then, with the arms in "Cross" position once more, bend the forward knee and touch the ground with the hand, at the same time keeping the other arm extended backward.

Reverse this.

This movement is also excellent for the muscles of the body and back.


Wall Balance (Ready-Bend!)

Stand sideways to the wall about two feet and a half away; now extend both arms in the "Cross" position, and then lift the foot that is farthest away from the wall and lean over until the extended fingers of the other hand touch the wall; push back into original position. Move out a little farther from the wall and repeat. Do this until the distance is as far as can comfortably be recovered by pushing the hand against the wall.

Reverse this exercise, so as to do it with the other arm.

This is an excellent workout for the shoulder muscles as well as for the forearms, and gives some exercise to the body.

## Stepping (Ready-Step!)

Standing erect at "Attention," step to the right with the right foot about six inches, merely touching the toe to the ground, and bring the foot back to the "Attention" position.

The object of this movement is to give control of the muscles of the leg in addition to the balancing of the body. Care should be taken to keep the body absolutely motionless while the exercise is in progress. The toe is only touched to the ground and the foot is brought immediately back into position.

This movement has a quieting effect after more violent exercising. It can be done either sideways, forward, or back.

## Running in Place (Mark Time - March!)

Beginning with "Marking Time!" Now raise the feet alternately from the ground, a little higher each time, until the knees come up practically to a level with the waist. Then perform this same motion on the toes and shift into a run while still holding the same position - that is, while going up and down on the toes. Men who have considerable weight around the waist-line should place their hands on the abdomen when performing this exercise.

Body-turning (Ready-Cross! Ready-Turn!)

This movement consists in turning the body at the hips while keeping the feet and legs in the original position. It may be done from almost any of the positions already outlined, and is moderate work for the muscles of the waist. Do it first with the arms in "Cross" position, turning to the right as far as possible; then back to the "Front," or original, position; then to the left as far as possible, and back to the "Front," or original, position, taking pains that the turning is executed above the hips while the legs and feet hold their original position. A more pronounced method is given in the "Daily Dozen" in "Wave" and "Weave."

Heel-raising (Ready-Rise!)

Standing on both feet at "Attention," raise the heels, and hold the position for a moment; then drop the heels again. Repeat this.

Now, standing in "Stride Position," go up onto the toes again. Drop the heels and repeat.

This is an excellent exercise for the muscles of the calf.

## GROUP EXERCISES

No. 1. Attention! (or "Hands!")

Hips: Same position, but hands on hips, elbows back.

Neck (or "Head"): Same position, but hands on back of neck, elbows back.

Cross: Same position, but arms extended full length out from body, palms down.

Grind: Maintaining the "Cross" position, turn palms up, and then make ten circles with hands, the diameter of the circle to be one foot (Fig. 12). In doing this keep the arms horizontally out from the body, and on the backward sweep try to make the shoulder-blades almost meet at the back. (See Fig. 4, Chapter XI.) Rest ten seconds. Deep breathing with hands on hips.


No. 2. Attention!

Stretch: Lift arms straight up above head, palms out.

Reach: Bring arms down, extending them straight out in front. Palms in, but keep shoulders back.

Fling: Bend elbows out and bring hands in to chest, palms down. Then to "Cross," back to "Fling" again, and so on ten times. (See Fig. 13.)

Wave: Assume "Reach" position. Now bend the arms sharply at wrists and just let the fingers interlock. Bring the inside of elbow close to head, keeping head up.

Then, by turning the body at the hips and keeping the back straight, cause the hands to make a complete circle of the diameter of a foot (Fig. 14). Do this five times, and then reverse for five times. (See Fig. 12, Chapter XIII.) Rest ten seconds. Then deep breathing, lifting arms on inhalations and crossing them on exhalations.

No. 3. Attention!

Stride: Separate the feet by taking a step to right, bringing the feet about eighteen inches apart.

Weave: Turn the body at the hips while keeping the arms horizontally extended and bending the right knee slightly. Bring the right hand down to the ground midway between the feet and let the left arm go up, keeping its horizontal position from the body, the spine doing the turning. Hold this position five seconds; then up to "Cross" position and turn the body the reverse way, bending left knee and bringing left hand to ground. Hold five seconds, then up. Repeat five times for each hand. (See Fig. 14, Chapter XIII.)

Curl: From "Cross" position, clench the fists and bring arms in slowly to the side and up into the armpits, at the same time bending the body and head backward (Fig. 15). The fists should be clenched and the wrists bent, bring the hands in toward the chest, the elbows out, and inhaling. (See Fig. 9, Chapter XII.)

Forward: From the above position, gradually bring the body up to an erect position, extending the hands to a "Reach" position, and slowly bend the body forward at the hips, exhaling at the same time, and letting the hands go back past the hips and as high behind the back as possible, keeping the head up and the eyes looking directly forward, not down. Go down about to the level of the wrist, then back to "Cross" position again, and repeat this backward and forward movement five times.

No. 4. Attention! (Cross-Crawl!) Assume the "Cross" position.

Crawl: While still keeping the neck back, the chin, and the chest arched, slowly lift the right hand and arm until it points directly upward, then curl in right arm over the head, at the same time dropping the left shoulder and sliding the left hand and arm down along the side of the left leg until the fingers reach directly to the knee, or as far as comfortable. Now come back from this position. (See Figs. 7 and 8, Chapter XII.) "Cross" once more and raise the other arm in similar fashion. Repeat this five times on each side.

No. 5. Attention! (Cross-Crouch!)

Crouch: Assume the "Cross" position of the arms and "Stride" stand, feet about eighteen inches apart. Now, keeping the head up and the neck back and back straight, bend the knees and come down slowly, not too far (Fig. 16), until fully accustomed to it, and up again. Repeat this five times. (See Fig. 10, Chapter XII.)

No. 6. Attention!

Heel-raising: Lift the heels from the floor, maintain the position on the toes for a second, then back onto the heels once more. Repeat some ten times, then take the

"Stride" stand and repeat ten times in this position.

No. 7. Attention!

Wing-work: Raise the arms to the "Cross." Then lift arms straight over head, inhaling; then, bending body forward and keeping the neck straight, swing the arms backward at the shoulder, exhaling, and come forward until the body is about level with the waist; then up again (Fig. 17). Picture the arms as looking like a bird's wings. Repeat this five times in each direction. (See Figs. 15, 15a, Chapter XIII.) Final deep breathing, with arm lifting as before.

FOOTNOTES:

[Footnote 1: This is the same movement as in the ordinary "Cross" position, except that the hands are kept clenched.]

# CHAPTER VI

## A TEN-DAY PROGRAM

### FIRST DAY

Attention!

Hips Firm
Neck Firm
Arms Bend
Arms Cross
Arms Stretch
Arms Reach
Mark Time
Mark Time on Toes

Attention!

Stepping
Heels Raise
Deep Breathing (At "Arms Stretch")

Hike or Outdoor Work

Walk half-mile on level, each man at his own stride.

Walk in pairs - column of twos; the shorter men should

be in front.


SECOND DAY

Attention!

Hips Firm
Neck Firm
Body Prone
Hips Firm
Stride Stand
Body Bend (Side to left and right)

Attention!

Arms Bend
Arms Cross
Balancing (On one foot - to right and left)
Arms Stretch
Mark Time
Mark Time on Toes

Attention!

Heels Raise
Stepping
Deep Breathing

Hike or Outdoor Work

Walk three-quarters of a mile, column of twos, keeping step. Starting at command, "Forward - March!" beginning with left foot. Leader calls "Company - Halt!" three or four times, and then "Forward - March!" again. Leader commands occasionally, "Change Step - March!"

## THIRD DAY

Attention!

Arms Bend
Arms Cross
Stride Stand
Turn Body (On hips - right and left)

Attention!

Neck Firm
Body Prone
Body Backward Bend

Attention!

Balancing (On one foot - to right and left)
Mark Time
Mark Time on Toes
Stride Stand
Heels Raise
Deep Breathing

Hike or Outdoor Work

Walk a mile, column of twos, keeping step. Last half-mile command men to stand up and keep their necks pressed back against their collars, chins in.


## FOURTH DAY

Attention!

Arms Bend

Arms Stretch
Palms Front
Bring Arms Downward and Backward

Attention!

Arms Bend
Arms Cross
Balancing (On one foot - to right and left)
Stride Stand (Foot advanced)
Bend Knee and Touch Floor with Hand (Right and left)
Mark Time
Mark Time on Toes
Stepping
Deep Breathing

Hike or Outdoor Work

Walk a mile, marching step, column of twos, shorter men in front, but try to get them up to a thirty-inch stride. Make a portion of the march slightly up-hill, and last half-mile with necks back, chin in, chest out.


FIFTH DAY

Attention!

Arms Bend
Arms Cross
Shoulder-grinding (Moving hands in circle and backward)

Attention!

Stride Stand

Arms Cross
Balancing (On one foot - to right and left)
Crouch (Quarter-bend)
Mark Time
Mark Time on Toes
Faster

Attention!

Stepping
Deep Breathing

Hike or Outdoor Work

Walk a mile and a quarter, column of twos. Insist on thirty-inch stride, but put shorter men in front. Make a little stiffer grade. No more talking in ranks. Insist upon necks back, chins in, and chests out all the way.


## SIXTH DAY

Attention!

Arms Bend
Arms Wing
Arms Fling
Arms Cross
Shoulder-grinding

Attention!

Stride Stand
Arms Cross
Balancing (On one foot - to right and left)
Body-turning

Crouch (Quarter-bend)

Attention!
Mark Time
Mark Time on Toes
Faster
Running in Place
Stepping
Deep Breathing

Hike or Outdoor Work

Bring men into company line and "count off." Explain "squad" formation. March mile and a quarter in column of squads. Take a stiffer grade. No talking in ranks. Keep to thirty-inch stride and give it a regular beat. No sloppiness. Make it a firm, steady march, and keep urging the men to breathe deeply and steadily.


SEVENTH DAY

Attention!

Right Face
Left Face
About Face
Repeat

Attention!

Balancing (On one foot - to right and left)
Stride Stand
Heel-raising
Body-bending Sideways
Mark Time

Mark Time on Toes
Faster
Running in Place
Stepping
 Deep Breathing

Hike or Outdoor Work

Company formation. Count off. "Squads Right - March!" Mile and a quarter. Silence in ranks. Erect carriage. Hips back. Deep breathing. Steady thirty-inch stride. Stiff incline. No lagging, but take it much the same as on the level. On the way, in some five minutes after the grade has been covered, give them "Double Time" for about twenty steps.

## EIGHTH DAY

Attention!

Right Face
Left Face
About Face
Repeat
Attention!

Arms Cross
Balancing (On one foot - to right and left)
Stride Stand
Crouch (Quarter-bend)

Attention!

Arms Cross
Arms Stretch

Palms Front
Bring Arms Downward and Backward
Mark Time
Mark Time on Toes
Faster
Running in Place
Stepping
Deep Breathing

Hike or Outdoor Work

Company formation. Count off. "Squads Right - March!" While marching explain to them "To the Rear - March," and have them do it three or four times. Distance mile and a half, with same hill work as before. Give them "Double Time" for twenty steps twice during the march.


NINTH DAY

Attention!

Forward - March (Three steps and come to "Attention!")
Same Steps Backward
Same Steps Sideways
Make Complete Square (Three steps forward, three to the right, three backward, and three to the left)
Hips Firm
Neck Firm
Body Prone
Body Backward Bend
Body Sideways Bend
Mark Time
Mark Time on Toes
Faster

Running in Place
Stepping
Deep Breathing
Hike or Outdoor Work

Get some bars of iron, one inch in diameter and three feet long. They should cost fifty cents apiece, and weigh about eight pounds. Give half the company these bars to carry, and at the middle of the hike transfer them to the other half to bring home. Distance mile and a half. No "Double Time." Carry the bars by the middle in the hands, and then for a time behind the back and through the elbows, with the hands in front.


TENTH DAY

Attention!

Arms Cross
Body and Knee Bend, turning on Hips and touching Floor with Hand
(First one and then the other. The right hand on bending right knee and the left hand on bending left knee).

Attention!

Hips Firm
Neck Firm
Body Prone
Body Backward Bend
Attention!

Stride Stand
Arms Cross
Balancing (On one foot - to right and left)

Crouch (Quarter-bend)

Attention!
Mark Time
Mark Time on Toes
Faster
Running in Place

Attention!

Stepping
Deep Breathing

Hike or Outdoor Work

Carry bars, distance mile and a quarter, every man carrying his bar all the way. "Double-time" them once during march for twenty steps. Insist on erect carriage all the way, with neck back against collars.

# PART II

# THE DAILY DOZEN

## A CONDENSED SYSTEM OF EITHER GROUP OR INDIVIDUAL SETTING-UP EXERCISES

# CHAPTER VII

We may now consider the question of time-saving for those who may be obliged to largely forego pleasurable exercise and who yet desire to keep fit and well in spite of this deprivation.

There are two divisions in this class, as may be shown in the case of the present world war. The first class embraces all the men in active service, with two subdivisions - officers who are over forty and officers and privates who are under that age. The second class comprises the men (and women, too, for that matter) who, unable to do service at the front, must support the troops in various ways behind the lines. It is said that it takes five men behind the line to support one man at the front, and, judging from the pressure that already has come upon our people, this is manifestly not an incorrect statement. These reserves must be kept in good physical condition, and with this end in view the writer has prepared a modified form of setting-up exercises which has been tested out with large numbers in actual practice.

These exercises are intended to prepare the younger men for the more strenuous training which they are to undergo later; in the case of the older men, they are to be used before entering upon the ordinary day of business routine. After a great deal of study a system has been devised which answers the needs in both cases; it is not too strenuous for the older men, and it will add suppleness, vitality, and endurance to the physical assets of the younger men.

## A MODERN PHYSICAL SYSTEM

We know how, in the stress of affairs brought about by war, not only individuals, but nations are suddenly awakened to the fact that what may have been good enough even a year ago is antiquated and out of date to-day. Under the pressure of war we are driven, whether we wish it or not, to put to immediate test virtually every fact of our daily lives. We find that almost every machine and well-nigh every method may be improved - in fact, that it must be improved.

Boats, aeroplanes, guns, industrial processes, even the actual business of living itself, all are being submitted to the test of emergency and are being made over upon new lines. So it is with our setting-up exercises. We can no longer afford to waste time or motion or effort. We are teaching on an intensive scale and we must take nothing out of a man in preparation; rather we must add to his store of vitality and energy. Perhaps we find that the routine of his ordinary work will strengthen sufficiently his legs and arms. This is astonishingly true. What we must now do is to supple him, to quicken his co-ordination, to improve his poise, and to put his trunk and thorax into better shape. We must give him endurance, quickness of response, and resistive force. This, therefore, being our problem, we eliminate the arm and leg exercises and go directly for the trunk and thorax. We must quicken co-ordination and improve the man's rapidity of response to command. And standing out above all is this major principle: "No vitality should be taken out of a man by these setting-up exercises; he should not be tired out, but rather made ready for the regular work of the day."

## OUT-OF-DATE IDEAS

This war in which we are engaged has brought to our people some all-compelling truths. And the greatest of these is that our men, the flower of our racial stock, are deficient physically when put to the test before examining-boards. When one sees some two thousand men examined by draft boards to secure two hundred men for our army, as happened in some cases, when one reads that in a physical examination for the sanitary police force in Cleveland thirty-seven out of forty-two women passed and only twenty-two men out of seventy-two, one is ready indeed to believe that we have failed to produce men who can be called upon when the need arises to defend our country.

Our athletic sports have produced the right spirit, as the rush of athletes to the service has shown. But our calisthenics, our general building-up exercises have apparently failed in the physical development of our youth. They are antique. Permit me to illustrate. Only recently Professor Bolen, the authority on Swedish exercises, died and left behind him the record of his work. After twenty-five years of study he had decided that setting-up exercises were unnecessary in the case of a man's legs or arms or pectoral muscles, and that the attention should be devoted to the trunk - that is, to the engine itself.

# OLD-TIME FALLACIES

Here is what was once considered to be a reasonable morning "setting-up" exercise, and which, if coupled with a five-mile rapid walk and hopping first on one foot and then on the other for a half-mile, would prepare a man for his day's work.

On rising, let him stand erect, brace his chest firmly out, and, breathing deeply, curl dumbbells (ten pounds each for a 165-pound man) fifty times without stopping. Then placing the bells on the floor at his feet, and bending his knees a little and his arms none at all, let him rise to an upright position with them fifty times.

After another minute's rest, standing erect, let him lift the bells fifty times as far up and out behind him as he can, keeping the elbows straight and taking care, when the bells reach the highest point behind, to hold them still there a moment.

Next, starting with the bells at the shoulders, let him push them up high over the head and lower them fifty times continuously.

Is it any wonder that we abandoned such "setting-up"?

Again, it was pointed out how, by special exercises, a man might increase his biceps two or three inches in a year and the calves of his legs an inch or two! Now what was the average man to do this for? What was the object? To admire himself in the mirror? Or did he intend to make of himself a professional weightlifter? Practically the only real good in all this was the deep breathing, and that would not be lasting except in so far as a part of the exercises tended to open up the chest. How many of us have heard that fairy-tale that if we practised deep breathing for a few minutes daily our lungs would acquire the habit and we should continue it unconsciously when seated at our desks!

## A PERFECTLY USELESS STUNT

Just to show what we are *not* attempting to do, here is a quotation illustrating perfectly the old-fashioned idea that health depends upon extraordinary muscular development:

> At our suggestion he began practising this simple raising and lowering of the heels. In less than four months he had increased the girth of each calf one whole inch. When asked how many strokes a day he averaged, he said that it was from fifteen hundred to two thousand, varied some days by his holding in each hand, during the process, a twelve-pound dumbbell, and then only doing one thousand or thereabouts. The time he found most convenient was in the morning on rising, and just before retiring at night. The work did not take much time; seventy strokes a minute was found a good ordinary rate, so that fifteen minutes at each end of the day was all he needed.

We new recognize how silly are such exercises taken for the mere sake of adding an inch or two to an already serviceable muscle.

## PENNY-WISE AND POUND-FOOLISH

It is poor gymnastics when the main object is to expend a certain number of foot-pounds of energy to secure increase in cardiac and pulmonary activity, without care being taken that these organs are in a favorable condition to meet the increased demand put upon them. It is poor gymnastics if we desire to astound the world by nicely finished and smoothly gliding combinations of complex movements fit to be put into the repertoire of a juggler, or by exhibitions of strength vying with those of a Sandow, if we do not take into consideration the effects upon the vital functions.

"Look at these fellows," said the physician, "built like giants and rotten inside!" True, he was speaking of a lot of big negroes, but he found the same condition in others - men with stiff muscles and slow movements, men with shoulders pulled forward and no chest expansion, breathing wholly with their abdomens. As he put it, "Those men will to-morrow be the recruits for another army, the one which fills the tuberculosis hospitals."

## NATURE'S PROCESS

What we want is suppleness, chest expansion, resistive force, and endurance; and these do not come from great bulging knots of muscle nor from extraordinary feats of strength. Rapid shifts from severe training to a life of ease and indulgence is not Nature's process. It is not the way in which she carries on her work. Every step she makes is a little one. She seems never to reckon time as an essential in her economy. We should heed the lesson. The man who eats, drinks, and neglects all care of himself for a year, and then rushes madly into a period of severe physical exercise and reduction, may at the end of the month, if he possesses sufficient vitality, come out feeling fine. But if he repeats the process of letting himself go, Nature puts on the fat more and more and a second severe reduction becomes necessary. And it is only a question of time as to the exhaustion of any man's vitality through these extremes.

## TIME THE GREAT ELEMENT

Any one who has had the opportunity of talking with the men in authority who are bearing the burden of fitting a nation for the present emergency cannot fail to be impressed with the fact that time is the great element. We must really prepare our men, we must make them fit in the shortest space of time that will accomplish the result. And we must conserve our man-power. It is no longer a question of putting on such severe work as shall weed out all but the physical giants; we are not trying (as seemed to be the idea in the first Plattsburg camps, before the war) to make the going so stiff as to leave us only 50 per cent. Of hardened men. We want every man who can be brought along rapidly into condition, and not the strongest only. Hence the problem takes on a new phase.

We all recognize that the quality and previous training of the men this country is sending into service have a very potent bearing upon the length of time required to make fighters of them. For, after all, the man whose training and discipline have been along a kindred line becomes serviceable much earlier than the man who has to acquire the necessary spirit and quality. No one who has listened to the coaches of our various college teams, or who has read either the preliminary prospects of a game or the account of it afterward, but must have been impressed with the continual repetition of emphasis upon the "fighting spirit."

Hence, when our athletes flock almost *en masse* to the colors, it means that we are enlisting a large number of picked men who have been in training both mentally and physically, and who, under discipline, will make obedient, courageous, and enthusiastic fighters. But a large number of these have been out of college or out of strenuous athletics a year or two, or longer, and they need physical conditioning to get back.

There is thus a new idea of considerable importance involved in these condensed setting-up exercises. For the world does move, and those who thought themselves up to date on boats, aeroplanes, drill, and the like have found even within a year that they must make acquaint-tance with advanced theories and new and improved methods.

## ESSENTIAL PRINCIPLES

Probably the most vital point is that the setting-up exercises should not "take it out of the men." If we find a man exhilarated and made eager to work at the end of his setting-up we have accomplished far more than if we tire him out or exhaust any of his store of vitality. If, in addition to this, we can reduce the amount of time occupied in these setting-up exercises and yet obtain results, we have saved that much more time for other work.

Because they did take it out of the men, the old-time

conventional setting-up exercises were shirked and the leaders were unable to detect this shirking; men went through the motions, but slacked the real work.

Furthermore, all these systems tended to take a longer period of time than was necessary to accomplish the desired results, and made "muscle bound" the men who practised them.

It has been found in sports and athletic games that over-developed biceps, startling pectoral muscles, and tremendously muscled legs are a disadvantage rather than an advantage. The real essential is, after all, the engine, the part under the hood, as it were - lungs, heart, and trunk. Finally, if we give a man endurance and suppleness he becomes more available in time of need.

Another point of equal importance is that the setting-up exercises should be rendered as simple as possible. If we are obliged to spend a considerable period of time in teaching the leader so that he can handle setting-up exercises, extension of the number of leaders is rendered increasingly difficult. If, therefore, we can make this leadership so simple that a long course of instruction is not necessary, we save here, in these days of necessarily rapid preparation, a very material amount of time.

Still, further, it is found that many of the present setting-up exercises made an extraordinarily wide variation of effort between heavy and light men. The light man would put in only a small amount of muscular effort, whereas the heavy man, in the same length of time and under the same exercise, would be taxed far more than he could comfortably stand.

Again, in the point of age, similar variations necessarily

exist. Naturally it is out of the question to assume that the youth from eighteen to twenty-five and the man of fifty-five to sixty can take the same amount and the same kind of exercise. On the other hand, if we consider the work each is required to do in his daily routine, we can, so far as the setting-up exercises are concerned, bring the two points nearer together, especially if we regard these setting-up exercises in the proper light - a mere preparation for the more onerous tasks that are to follow.

## MODERN PHYSICAL EDUCATION

Bearing all these points in mind, we test out the setting-up exercises so that we may obtain a set answering the following requirements:

First - Reduce them to a period of eight or ten minutes once or twice a day.

Second - Make them simple for leaders to learn.

Third - Eliminate movements that, on account of the daily work, are unnecessary.

Fourth - Render them more difficult of evasion or shirking.

Fifth - Direct them specifically in the line of increased resisting power, endurance, and suppleness.

Sixth - Make them of value in establishing co-ordination, muscular control, and more prompt response to command.

Seventh - Equalize them for use by both heavy and light men.

Eighth - Select the exercises in such a way that the set may be of nearly equal value to both enlisted men and officers, as well as to executives behind the lines.

## SLACKING IN SETTING-UP DRILLS

Many of us have seen setting-up drills of various kinds. Moving pictures of such drills show in a very striking way how much of the work not only could be slacked, but *is* being slacked right along. In fact, high officers in our service have become so disgusted with the setting-up exercises as to consider abandoning them altogether. In some stations or cantonments a great many men were tired out with the setting-up exercises; so much so that they had neither life nor vitality for some little time for other work. For the sake of illustration, let us examine one particular movement. It consists of the men lying flat on the ground or floor; then, with straight back, lifting themselves by the arms; finally, giving a jump with the arms and clapping the hands together once, and then coming back to the original position. The non-commissioned officer who was leading this exercise weighed about 138 pounds. It is easy to imagine the contrast between his doing this stunt and a heavy man of 180 or 190 pounds attempting it.

It is unnecessary to describe in detail the parts of the setting-up exercise which tend to develop members which are already pretty thoroughly exercised in the daily routine of work and drill. The average man of the service needs expansion of chest capacity, which adds to his resistive power; a stronger, better-developed back;

and suppleness and quickness and mobility of trunk. To develop these qualities we must have exercises which may be continued on board ship or near the front, and which can be carried on without apparatus.

The ordinary system of setting-up exercises has been growing out of favor for some time. Athletic trainers have come to look with considerable suspicion upon the gymnasium-made candidate with big biceps and large knots of muscles. It was also found that, outside of weight-lifting and inordinate "chinning" and apparent great strength on the parallel bars, these men were not so valuable as the lesser muscled but more supple candidates. To put it briefly, it was found in actual practice that what was under the ribs was of more value than what lay over them.


## A CALL FOR WORK THAT WILL COUNT

Even at the risk of repetition, some facts should be driven home.

We are now working under conditions that should especially emphasize the fact of time-saving. We must take ourselves seriously, whether we are in the lines or behind the lines.

In the eight million men in this country between the ages of forty-five and sixty-four are the country's greatest executives and financiers. We can no longer give these executives and financiers two months in the South in the winter and a long summer vacation. We can no longer let a Plattsburg camp be a strenuous sifting out, a mere survival of the physically fittest. We need every man whom we can make available, and we need him with his vitality fully preserved and his endurance appreciably heightened. Some are stronger, naturally, than others. In football parlance we are no longer trying to pick a team out of a squad of two hundred men; we are trying to get a hundred and seventy-five out of the two hundred that can stand a fair pace and have enough left to fight with when they get there. Any one who has been in touch with affairs in Washington, any one who has been engaged in our munition-plants and in our factories, any one who has worked upon Liberty Bond drives or Red Cross fund-raising, knows that if we are to support our boys on land and sea, these men who are trying to solve the problems of executive management, and who have the task of raising funds in thousandfold increased volume, must be also carefully conserved. For, after all, even though we spell Patriotism with a capital P and Government with a capital G, even though army and navy orders take precedence, there is one great mistress of all, Dame Nature! And when she taps a man on the shoulder and says, "Quit!" that man stops; and when he offers the excuse that he has done it out of patriotism and loyalty she merely says: "I don't care why you did it, you have finished!" And there is no appeal to Washington from her verdict.

## THE BIG PROBLEM

We shall soon hear the call for more men, men to fight and men to support the men who fight. The game is on. We are all in it now, either on the field or on the side-lines. We need to train for it fast and we have no time to waste. For, after all, it is condition that tells. It is the man who can stay, who can work at highest efficiency, and who can hold out the longest who is going to be most valuable. If we save even ten minutes a day in the setting-up exercises, we save, with a hundred thousand men, 16,666 hours daily toward perfecting their other knowledge. If we can make an able officer or a competent executive last a year longer or even six months under the increased strain, it gives us a year or six months more in which his understudy can gather the necessary experience to take up his task.

Millions of our youth are going out to fight, but disease and exhaustion will kill more of them than will the guns of the enemy. Thousands of men of the best brain-power in this country are going into committee-rooms and conferences every day from nine in the morning till twelve at night to devise better and more efficacious means of stopping the progress of the Hun. If these men's brains are of value, and we know they are, then the more clearly they act and the longer they last, the better for the country.

## THE NEED FOR A CONDENSED SYSTEM OF CALISTHENICS

The demonstration, with a group of busy business executives and professional men, of the possibility of physical fitness at a small expenditure has been already mentioned. This idea has spread and many units of the Senior Service Corps have been organized. The writer's services were later on drafted into national work. At the call of the Secretary of the Navy, he was asked to take a position on the Naval Commission to develop athletic sports and games and physical fitness in our men at the various naval stations. In one week alone requests came from over four hundred communities to establish units of this work among business and professional men. Finding that it was impossible to answer all these calls, the writer devoted himself personally to a class in Washington, consisting of several Cabinet members, officials of the Federal Reserve Board, and others, and these men profited extremely from the work. But this should be done on a far larger scale.

The Hon. Daniel C. Roper, who was a member of the original class in Washington, requested the writer to come down and spend a month or six weeks in Washington, to organize drill groups in the various departments, several of them, like the Department of the Interior, having received requests to the number of three hundred or four hundred from men who wished to make themselves better fit physically for the work of these strenuous days. This, together with the demands from so many communities throughout the country, show that we are all now awake to the necessity of this cardinal feature of the nation's welfare, the physical fitness and stamina of its youth and men. This new gospel cannot be spread by one individual missionary, although there is little doubt that, wherever the story is told, thousands of our overworked and under-exercised men are glad to avail themselves of the opportunity.

This is the reason why the author has been led to devise a set of exercises that can be put in small compass, as regards both instruction and time required. Here follows a brief syllabus of the plan, in the hope of placing it within reach of men who can afford but little time for anything outside of their pressing office duties. We can no longer take delightful vacations of indefinite length to restore our waning vitality. The country needs every man and needs him at the best of his power.

## A REASONABLE PROGRAM

No matter how driven a man may be, it seems only reasonable to think that he should be able to spend ten minutes twice a day on a condensed system, or setting-up exercise, adding to it an outdoor walk of half an hour. By this means he can keep himself physically fit to bear the burdens which are falling more and more heavily upon the shoulders of us all. The men who are going to the front first should have every chance of conserving their vitality and increasing their resistive forces. Those of us who must do work behind the lines should be kept equally fit for that larger work without which the machine must inevitably break down. The method is scientific and it has been tested on men of all ages from eighteen to seventy. It embodies the elimination of all wasted effort and concentration upon points of approved and essential worth. It is as much a man's duty to make himself fit and to keep himself in that condition as it is to carry on any other part of his work. This method should be adopted not only in every department at Washington, but throughout the country; it should be taught in our schools and colleges, and so thoroughly that never again in a world-wide crisis shall we find ourselves physically unprepared.

WALTER CAMP

# CHAPTER VIII

Vacillation and doubt are poison to the nerves.

This is the reason why it is advisable to teach co-ordination, prompt response to the command of the brain over the muscles, and the general sense of self-control which comes to a man when he has only to think in order to turn that thought into quick action. One of the penalties of the executive position is that, although the man begins as a disciplined private, when he goes up higher and gradually reaches the point where he gives commands only, and never has any practice in obeying them, he gets the habit of pushing buttons to make other people jump, while there are no buttons pushed to make him jump.

## WORRY AND FEAR

Now as to worry. It has been said, and not untruly, that one of the very largest causes of worry is bodily weakness. And in more than a majority of cases this weakness comes from poor physical condition. A good digestion and proper elimination seem to make the organism move smoothly, not alone with muscles, but with nerves. Hence if we get the engine right, the lungs doing their duty, the skin acting as it should, and the bowels and kidneys taking off the waste products, we generally find a robust man, little given to that most expensive habit, "worry."

Fear is the forerunner of illness.

There is nothing quite so effective in producing a bad condition of the human system as fear, and this fear is what worry develops into; later it becomes pure, downright cowardice.

Worry makes cowards. If a man has enough worry and anxiety, fear follows in its wake, and then the man becomes a mental and moral and often a physical coward.


## THE FATAL MISTAKE

The average man, when he is pressed to overwork, thinks that by cutting out some of his exercise and devoting that extra time to his work he can accomplish more. There never was a greater mistake; in the long run this method is the most expensive of all. No factory manager would think of running his automatic machines twice as long with half the amount of oil, and yet that is just what the man is trying to do in this case. The result is that he gradually piles up the various toxic products within himself until self-poisoning is inevitable. All his organs struggle to eliminate these poisons, but, being given no assistance, they gradually become less and less efficient, and then begins the payment of the penalty, for Nature never forgives this kind of treatment. From a practical, useful running machine he retrogrades into something fit only for the scrap-heap. The history is the same in all cases, although it may be more or less prolonged. The discomfort, occasional slight illnesses, the gradual loss of effective thought and power to concentrate, lack of appetite, unreasonable temper, insomnia, nerve diseases, and perhaps a complete nervous and physical breakdown if the conditions are not recognized in time, are the varying punishments inflicted by Nature.

I have referred to Nature's order, "You must earn your bread by the sweat of your brow." Almost every one, in these modern days of civilization, is earning his bread in some other way; well, he must make up for this by some kind of exercise or else Nature will surely take her toll. When men were earning their bread by the sweat of their brows they were not always sure of getting a surplus of it, and that was not a half-bad thing. In fact, it was far better for the race than present conditions under which so many men have given up physical work altogether. But instead of cutting down on their food they double up on it.

## SOMETHING OUT OF A BOTTLE

The usual temporary panacea for these ills of the flesh is to get some so-called "specific" in the form of a medicine and gobble it religiously. Thousands of men and women, who are unwilling to take five or ten minutes' exercise two or three times a day, will swallow something out of a bottle on a spoon before each meal, with a splendid satisfaction and confidence. Perhaps temporarily it produces improved results. At any rate, it gives a sense of mental satisfaction, and that something stands off the trouble for a while. There is still another method which has some show of reason in it, although, after all, it does not compare with the wiser, saner course. A man or woman is persuaded that if he or she will only give up some particularly attractive self-indulgence the result will be increased health and vigor. For instance, there is a common belief that tea or coffee is the cause of many ills. Perhaps this is true, but the giving up of tea or coffee will never cure the ills that come from lack of exercise, loss of fresh air, over-eating, and over-indulgence. The mere fact that a person is giving up something that he likes does not make him immune to the penalties which he incurs day after day by other offenses against the laws of Nature.

## CONSERVING THE PRESIDENT'S HEALTH

Rear-Admiral Carey T. Grayson, personal physician and health director to President Wilson, says:

"You may make the statement, in so many words, that physical exercise has been the means of making a normal, physically perfect man of the President. And when a man is in a normal condition he is in perfect health and physical trim. That was the initial intention in this case, just to make the President physically fit, and to keep him so."

Richard M. Winans says:

"The Admiral told me that when he first took charge of the President, Mr. Wilson was not a little averse to taking any sort of exercise. However, Doctor Grayson early succeeded in impressing upon Mr. Wilson that good health was an absolutely important factor in dealing with the grilling duties which would face him during the coming four years, and that his physical well-being was vital not only to himself, but to the welfare of the entire country."

The President has a dislike almost akin to abhorrence for mechanical appliances intended to exercise the muscles of the body. There is not a dumbbell, or an Indian club, nor a medicine-ball, nor a punching-bag, nor a turning-bar, nor a trapeze, nor a lifting or pulling apparatus, nor a muscle - exercising machine of any sort or description in the White House. The only mechanical device used by the President is a simple, unoffending golf-club.

Aside from his work in the open air, Mr. Wilson takes a number of physical exercises indoors, very few of which have ever been described in print. Some of these exercises are taken as a substitute for outdoor recreations at times when weather conditions are too extreme. But the major part of them, and especially the more unusual of these exercises, are regularly practised as a part of his daily routine. As a matter of fact, they are pretty closely dove-tailed in with his office work.

## FLEXING EXERCISES

However, if the President really has a favorite among his various physical exercises, it is said to be that of "flexing." This he employs almost entirely as an indoor exercise, and it perhaps is the one he practises more often than any other.

"Flexing," as Doctor Grayson put it into its simplest every-day term, is nothing more nor less than just good, old-fashioned "stretching" expressed in a scientific and systematized form of exercise. It is the most generally and commonly executed muscular exercise, and it is practised by nearly all the animal kingdom.

President Wilson uses his flexing movements with a

careful regard to system, and a great deal more regularly and frequently than any other of his varied physical exercises. Particularly during his periods of concentration, when at work at his desk in the preparation of his messages to Congress or in the drafting of notes to foreign governments, the President, at short intervals, will either settle back in his chair and flex his arms and hands and the muscles across his back and chest, or he will rise and stand erect for a more thorough practice of the flexing movements for a period of a minute or more. At these times he will throw his body into almost every conceivable posture - twisting, turning, bending, stooping, the arms down, forward, back, and over his head, the muscles of the limbs and entire body flexed almost to the point of tremor, the fingers spread, and the muscles rigidly tensed.

In the opinion of Doctor Grayson, if business and professional men, particularly those who work at high tension in the cities, would pause in their work at frequent intervals during the day and give a few seconds of their time to the energetic practice of the flexing or stretching exercises, there would soon come to be not only less, but, possibly in time, no cases reported of this or that noted man, the famous lawyer, merchant, or financier, dropping dead at his desk or in his home or in the street, on account of apoplexy caused by hardened arteries.

One of Mr. Wilson's principal physical movements is that of body-twisting. With the toes at a slight outward angle, the heels touching and the body erect, he begins the movement by twisting the body a little more than half-way around; then swinging back in an arc, at the same time bending at the hips, until he has completed the circle and reached a hip-bending position, with the fingers of one hand touching the floor, the other extended vertically. This gives a stretching movement to all of the muscles of the torso, side, back, and abdomen, as well as considerable play to the muscles of the legs and arms.

## THE UNPLEASANT SELF-AWAKENING

We as a nation, through the revelation of the draft, have been suddenly thrown upon the public screen as physically deficient. And that, too, when the echoes of the Eagle screaming over successes in the world Olympic games had hardly done sounding in our satisfied ears. Naturally, we don't like it. Deep down in our consciousness we are not only dissatisfied with the picture, but we feel that somehow it is distorted; we are hoping to prove that even a photograph does not always tell the truth, at least not the whole truth. Yet in this search for the truth there are some facts that we must face and admit. The first of these is that as a race - blended, if you please, but still the people of a nation - we are ambitious and hurried. We act a great deal more than we think. Cricket is too slow for us; only baseball has the fire and the dash we like. We haven't quite enough time even for that, and so we begin to leave the stands before the game is over, craning our necks as we walk along toward the exits for a last glimpse, and then rushing madly to get on the first car out. All this is typical of our life. We have had a measure of benefit from our athletics. They are a spur toward physical development as long as they last. But no sooner are school-days drawing to an end than we begin the mad rush - toward what? To see how fast we can make money or name or position. We take a final look backward at the last inning of these sports of ours, and then we rush out into the world of American hustle. The lucky ones prolong their playtime a little by a college course, but they, too, finally abandon sport in favor of business and let themselves go slack until they lose condition. A week or two in the summer, a fort-night's orgy of exercise, and then back to the grind of factory or desk. How can this way of living keep even a young man fit? Golf has been a godsend to the older man whose pocket-book can stand it, but what about the youth? And when pressure comes on the older man he quickly gives up his golf at the demand of business.

## WHY MEN DON'T KEEP FIT

Men who have really kept themselves fit are few. Those who have conscientiously started in to do this and then abandoned it are a host. There are valid reasons for this lamentable state of affairs.

First - Because the antiquated systems under which these men have attempted the task have

(1) Occupied too much time;
(2) Left men tired instead of refreshed;
(3) Exercised muscles which get all they need in a man's ordinary  pursuits.

Secondly - Because the instructors who have taught these systems have laid stress upon

(1) Mere increase in size of the muscles;
(2) Ability to do "stunts" which are of no practical use to a man;
(3) Unnecessary use of apparatus.

Thirdly - Because they made necessary the services of a teacher to

(1) Lead the exercises;
(2) Keep track of their number and variety;
(3) Give special treatment to produce results.

But these mistakes are in the past. Let us look toward a brighter, saner, and more productive future.

# CHAPTER IX

The following chapters give a set of exercises carefully tested upon thousands of men, and these exercises will be fully explained so that any individual reader may practise them daily and secure their full benefit. To each chapter are appended a few health hints, couched in language that is brief and to the point, in order that they may be readily remembered. The object is to make an efficient working-machine of the man without useless effort, to increase that man's resistive force against disease, to add to his suppleness and endurance, to give him poise and balance, and to develop co-ordination or control over his muscles. By doing this his power to work will be augmented, and at the same time any work that he does will be accomplished more readily and with less effort. Finally his cheerfulness will be increased, and those who work with him or under him or about him will be spared the disagreeable experiences that accompany association with a man whose irritability and irascibility have become part of his daily habit.

## A SHORTHAND METHOD

We call this system the "Daily Dozen Set-up." It is a shorthand system of setting-up exercises for use on any and all occasions.

The "Daily Dozen Set-up" consists of twelve exercises which, for ease in memorizing, are divided into four groups of three exercises each. Each exercise or movement is given a name, and the names of all the movements of a group commence with the same letter, thus:

GROUP I  GROUP II GROUP III GROUP IV

1. Hands 4. Grind  7. Crawl  10. Wave
2. Hips  5. Grate  8. Curl  11. Weave
3. Head  6. Grasp  9. Crouch 12. Wing

These exercises are not difficult nor exhausting, and do not demand great strength for their proper execution. They are designed, both from a scientific and a practical point of view, to give exactly the right amount of exercise to every muscle of the body. They are intended to promote suppleness, and especially to strengthen those muscles which are seldom brought into play in ordinary daily life. A conscientious fifteen minutes a day with the "Daily Dozen" will soon do more for a man than any amount of skilled physical feats or "strong-man stunts." When one first practises these movements their effect will be felt on the little-used muscles of the neck, back, and stomach; yet they will not leave the pronounced muscular fatigue which follows the ordinary exercises and which does more harm than good.

## HEALTH MAXIMS

Dress to be cool when you walk and warm when you ride.

Clean skin, clean socks, clean underwear every day.

Getting mad makes black marks on the health.

Sleep woos the physically tired man; she flouts the mentally exhausted.

Nature won't stand for overdrafts any more than your bank.

In a squad it is the job of each individual to make himself fit, for it is his example that helps the rest.

The leader may be no better than you, but some one must give the orders and set the pace.

Two things are essential to a clean skin; one is bathing and a rub-down, but the other is still more important, and that is perspiration.

Food, water, and oxygen are the fuel for running the human machine.

You never saw a dog fill his mouth with food and then take a drink to wash it down.

# CHAPTER X

Any setting-up exercises should be preparatory - that is, they should make men ready for the serious work of their day, and in no way exhaust any portion of their vitality. This modern "shorthand" method of setting-up leaves men in an exhilarated condition, and, instead of taking anything out of them, it prepares the body for any kind of work that may be required.

Each exercise starts from the position of "Attention," which is thus described in the army manual:

Heels on the same line and as near each other as the conformation of the man permits.

Feet turned out equally and forming with each other an angle of about sixty degrees.

Knees straight without stiffness.

The description of this exercise is the same as that given for the military command of "Attention," and the following points should be carefully noted:

It is not difficult to acquire a certain amount of accuracy in this position, but one of the easiest ways of getting men to assume it properly is to tell them to push their necks back. This seems more effective than to speak of holding the chin in with the head erect, or anything of that kind. If a man stands naturally and then forces the back of his neck back against his collar, he comes into very nearly the desired position of "Attention" so far as his head and neck are concerned.

The shoulders should be rolled a little downward and back, for that is the sensation which comes when one speaks of the shoulders being square. The chest should be arched and the abdomen drawn in somewhat. The effect is that of a man standing erect and feeling himself a little taller than usual.]

Body erect on hips, inclined a little forward; shoulders square and falling equally.

Arms and hands hanging naturally, backs of the hands outward; thumbs along the seams of the trousers; elbows near the body.

Head erect and straight to the front, chin slightly drawn in without constraint, eyes straight to the front. (See Fig. 1.)

Each movement, with the exception of the "Speed Test" (a catch exercise with which any man may test his rapidity of action and co-ordination), should be executed in a slow and measured manner. These exercises do not depend upon snap for their effect, but upon the steady, deliberate, but not extreme stretching of the muscles. Any tendency toward hurried, careless execution should be avoided in favor of uniformity of movement.

## GROUP I

Hands: This is the same position as "Attention." (See Fig. 1.)

The position called "Hips" is that of "Attention" with the hands placed on the hips, the fingers forward and the thumbs back, at the same time keeping the shoulders and elbows well back.]

Especial care should be taken to see that whenever, throughout the exercises, this position is taken - as at the completion of each movement - full control is retained over the arms; the hands should not be allowed to slap against the sides audibly.

It is not difficult to acquire a certain amount of accuracy in this position, but one of the easiest ways of getting men to assume it properly is to tell them to "push their necks back." This seems more effective than to speak of holding the chin in with the head erect, or anything of that kind. If a man stands naturally and then forces the back of his neck back against his collar, he comes into very nearly the desired position of "Attention," so far as his head and neck are concerned.

The shoulders should be rolled a little downward and back, for that is the sensation which comes when one speaks of the shoulders being square. The chest should be arched and the abdomen drawn in somewhat. The effect is that of a man standing erect and feeling himself a little taller than usual.

Hips: The hands are placed on the hips, with shoulders, elbows and thumbs well back. (See Fig. 2.) The position of "Hips" is that of "Attention" with the hands placed on the hips, the fingers forward and the thumbs back, at the same time keeping the shoulders and elbows well back.

Head: The hands are placed behind the neck, index finger-tips just touching and elbows forced back. (See Fig. 3.)

In the position called "Head" the body is still in the position of "Attention," the neck pushed well back, the fingers and the hands just touching behind the neck, and the elbows not allowed to push forward but kept as far back as the shoulders.]

In the position called "Head" the body is still in the position of "Attention," the neck pushed well back, the fingers and the hands just touching behind the neck, and the elbows not allowed to push forward but kept as far back as the shoulders.

Speed Test: The above three exercises, "Hands, Hips, Head," should be executed but a few times each, being preparatory to the "Speed Test." For this the pupil should concentrate his thought on running through the above set as rapidly as possible, at the same time making each position correct.

HEALTH MAXIMS

Success comes from service.

Don't make excuses. Make good.

If you feel tired, remember so does the other man.

After a hearty meal, stand up straight for fifteen minutes.

Your squad is only as good as the poorer ones. Don't be one of those.

The success of the drill depends upon the concentration of each man of the squad.

If you have a stake in life, it is worth playing the game for all there is in it.

The man who gets things is the one who pulls up his belt a hole tighter and goes out after them.

If you will save your smoke till after luncheon, you'll never have smoker's heart.

A bath, cold if you please, hot if you must, with a good rub, starts the day right.

# CHAPTER XI

## GROUP II

Grind: (The order is "Shoulder Grind. Ready - Cross. Balance Turn. Grind!") Assume the "Cross"[2] position. (See Fig. 2, Chapter V.) The palms are then turned up, with the backs of the hands down and the arms forced back as far as possible. (See Fig. 4.)

In the "Grind" special precaution should be taken not to let the center of the circle, that the hands are making, come in front of the shoulders; an attempt should almost be made to make the shoulder-blades meet. This is particularly necessary on the reverse.]

Then to a measured counting - "One, two, three, four, five," up to ten - circles of twelve-inch diameter are described with the finger tips, the latter moving forward and upward, the arms remaining stiff and pivoting from the shoulders. On the backward movement of the circle the arms should be forced back to the limit. A complete circle should be described at each count. Then reverse, going through the same process, the circles being described in the opposite direction.

In the "Grind" exercises special precaution should be taken not to let the center of the circle, that the hands are making, come in front of the shoulders; it should be straight out in the horizontal position; moreover, as the arm goes backward an attempt should be made to make the shoulder-blades almost meet. This is particularly necessary on the reverse - that is, when the hands are coming forward - for here the tendency, unless men keep the shoulders back, is to contract the chest.

Grate: (The order is "Shoulder Grate. Ready - Cross. Grate!") Assume the "Cross" position. Then at a count of "One" the arms are slowly raised, as a deep inhalation is taken, to an angle of forty-five degrees from horizontal; at the same time the heels are raised till the weight of the body rests on the balls of the feet. (See Fig. 5.)

The caution in the "Grate" position is not to let the arms drop, even a fraction of an inch, below the horizontal, and not to let them go up above the angle of forty-five degrees, for in either of these cases there is a distinct rest given to the shoulder muscles. Most of the ordinary exercises of this kind carry the arms above the head; this always releases the effort of the shoulder muscle and is therefore nearly valueless as an exercise for these members.

Another fault in this exercise is letting the head come forward. The neck should be kept back all the time.]

At "Two" the arms are slowly returned to "Cross" as all air is exhaled and the heels are lowered to a normal position. Care should be taken to see that the arms are not allowed to drop below the level of the shoulders or to rise more than forty-five degrees. The arms should be raised and lowered ten times.

The caution in the "Grate" position is not to let the arms

drop, even a fraction of an inch, below the horizontal, and not to let them go up above the angle of forty-five degrees, for in either of these cases there is a distinct rest given to the shoulder muscles. Most of the ordinary exercises of this kind carry the arms above the head; this always releases the effort of the shoulder muscle and is therefore nearly valueless as an exercise for these members.

Another fault in this exercise is letting the head come forward. The neck should be kept back all the time.

Grasp: (The order is "Head Grasp. Ready - Cross. Grasp!") Assume the "Cross" position. Then place the hands behind the head. With head up and eyes front, and in time with the counting, "One, two, three, four," the body is bent forward from the waist as far as possible. (See Fig. 6.)

In the "Grasp" position it is not necessary to go to extremes on the backward movement; only so far as is really comfortable. In the forward movement the body should come down practically at right angles to the hips, but the head should not be allowed to drop forward. The head should be kept up, with the elbows back and the eyes looking to the front.]

The body is returned to the upright in the same number of counts, and at an unusually slow "One" it is bent as far back as comfortable only from the waist, being returned to the upright at "Two." Care should be taken to see that this motion is slow and not jerky. The entire movement should be repeated five times.

In the "Grasp" position it is not necessary to go to an extreme on the backward movement; only so far as is really comfortable. In the forward movement the body should come down practically at right angles to the hips, but the head should not be allowed to drop forward. The head should be kept up, with the elbows back and the eyes looking to the front.

## HEALTH MAXIMS

Vacillation and doubt are poison to the nerves.

Fear is the forerunner of illness.

"Eyes in the boat" is as good a maxim at drill as in a shell.

When drinking a glass of water stand erect and take a full breath first; then drink with chest out and hips back and head up.

The men who chase the golf-ball don't have to pursue the doctor.

Two hours of outdoor exercise by the master never yet made him over-critical of the cook.

Nature never punished a man for getting his legs tired. She has punished many for getting their nerves exhausted.

The best record in golf is the record she has made of restored health to the middle-aged.

See how high you can hold your head and deeply you can breathe whenever you are out of doors.

Six to eight glasses of water a day, none with meals, will make you free of doctors.


FOOTNOTES:

[Footnote 2: On the "Cross" position, the arms should be straight out horizontally from the body, with the elbows locked. At the same time every resistance should be placed against the head and neck coming forward at all. These should be held in exactly the same position as at "Attention." The tendency is either to let the arms bend a little, or to let them drop a little below the horizontal, or even to hold them slightly above the level.]

# CHAPTER XII

## GROUP III

Crawl: (The order is "Crawl. Ready - Cross. Crawl!")
Assume the "Cross" position. The left palm is then
turned up, and on a count of "One, two, three, four" the
left arm is raised and the right arm is lowered laterally
until at "Four" the right arm should be in a position of
"Hands," while the left arm should be extended straight
up, with the palm to the right. (See Fig. 7.)

In the "Crawl" position it is not necessary, in the
beginning of the exercise, to slide the hand down the hip
any farther than is perfectly comfortable. But this
distance should be gradually increased, and it will be
found quite easy to do this as the muscles of the side
become more and more supple.]

Then on the count of "One, two, three, four" the body is
slowly bent sideways from the waist, the right hand
slipping down the right leg to or beyond the knee, and
the left arm bending in a half-circle over the head until
the fingers touch the right ear. (See Fig. 8.) At "Four"
the position of "Cross" is quickly resumed, and at "Two"
of the next counting the right palm is turned up and the
exercise is completed in the opposite direction.

In the "Crawl" position it is not necessary, in the

beginning of the exercise, to slide the hand down the hip any farther than is perfectly comfortable. But this distance should be gradually increased, and it will be found quite easy to do this as the muscles of the side become more and more supple.

Curl: (The order is "Curl. Ready - Cross. Curl!") Assume the "Cross" position. In this movement, at "Cross" the feet are spread until the heels are about twelve inches apart. The left foot remains stationary, the right foot being moved to accomplish this. On a count of "One, two, three, four," at the same time inhaling slowly, the fists and lower arms are bent down from the elbows, which are kept pressed back, and the fists are slowly curled up into the armpits. This position should be reached at "Three," when the head and shoulders should be forced back rather strongly, reaching the limit of motion at "Four." (See Fig. 9.) Again on the count of "One, two, three, four," at "One" the arms are extended straight forward from the shoulders, with the palms down, and exhalation is begun.

In the "Curl" position the head and shoulders should be thrown well back and the fists should go well up into the armpits. Keep the elbows back so that the entire thorax is lifted forward and up; at the same time take a deep inhalation.]

At "Two" the arms begin to fall and the body bends forward from the waist, head up and eyes front, until, at "Four," the body has reached the limit of motion and the arms have passed the sides and have been forced back and up (as the trunk assumes a horizontal position) as far as possible. At this point the abdomen should be well drawn in at the finish of exhalation.

(Note that in this figure the feet are together, an incorrect position for this exercise.) For a third time, on a count of "One, two, three, four" the body is straightened, reaching an upright position, with arms straight forward at "Three." "Cross" is assumed at "Four." As the body is straightened from the "Wing" position, a full breath should be taken, the lungs being filled, slowly, to the maximum as "Curl" is finally reached. This breath should be retained and then exhaled as the "Wing" position is taken. Inhale through the nose.

The entire movement should be repeated five times.

In the "Curl" position the head and shoulders should be thrown well back and the fists should go well up into the armpits. Keep the elbows back so that the entire thorax is lifted forward and up; at the same time take a deep inhalation.

Crouch: (The order is "Crouch. Ready - Cross. Crouch!") Assume the "Cross" position. In this movement, at "Cross" the feet are spread until the heels are about twelve inches apart. The left foot remains stationary, the right foot being moved to accomplish this. On a count of "One" the knees are bent, and, with the weight on the toes, the body is lowered nearly to the heels, keeping the trunk as nearly erect as possible. (See Fig. 10.)

The "Crouch" is intended for the acquisition of balance and poise, but is also good exercise for the legs. The back is kept straight and the balance preserved throughout.]

This is done at "One," and at "Two" the upright position is resumed.

The entire movement should be repeated ten times.

The "Crouch" position is intended for the acquisition of balance and poise; at the same time it is good exercise for the legs. The back should be kept straight and the balance preserved as the body goes up and down. This will be a little difficult at first, but will soon become natural.

## HEALTH MAXIMS

Worry makes cowards.

Happiness comes from health, not from money.

Co-operation with others is the life of the squad.

Drill is a mental as well as a physical discipline.

Work will take your mind off most of your ills.

Obesity comes from overloading the stomach and underworking the body.

Nine-tenths of the "blues" come from a bad liver and lack of outdoor exercise.

Wearing the same weight underclothing the year around will save you a lot of colds.

Your nose, not your mouth, was given you to breathe through.

Short shoes and shoes that don't fit cost a lot in the

long run.

Blood pressure does not come to the men who walk a lot out of doors; instead it looks for those who sit and eat a lot indoors.

Two men in an eight-oared shell may be able to go faster than the other six, but they never win the race that way.

# CHAPTER XIII

## GROUP IV

Wave: (The order is "Wave. Ready - Cross. Arms up. Wave!") Assume the "Cross" position. The arms are then stretched straight above the head, the fingers interlaced and the arms touching the ears. (See Fig. 11.)

On a count of "One, two, three, four" a complete circle, of about twenty-four inches in diameter, is described with the hands, the body bending only at the waist. The trunk should be bent as far backward as forward, and as far to one side as to the other. (See Fig. 12.)

In the "Wave" the tendency is to go too far forward and not far enough back, the result being an unsymmetrical motion. It is very easy to go forward, but more difficult to make the motion to the side and back. Care should be taken that the arms are kept squarely against the ears. The motion should be like waving the mast of a ship, the hips representing the deck and the trunk, head, and arms up to the top of the hands, the mast.]

The body should be forward at "One," to the right at "Two," backward at "Three," and to the left at "Four." The motion should be steady and not in jerks.

At "Reverse" the same movement should be repeated in

the opposite direction - i.e. to the left.

As the movement is completed for the fifteenth time the body should be brought to an erect position, stretching the arms up as far as possible; and at "Rest" the arms should drop slowly, laterally, to a "Hands" position. Five circles should be described in each direction.

In the "Wave" the tendency is to go too far forward, and not far enough back, the result being an unsymmetrical motion. It is very easy to go forward, but more difficult to make the motion to the side and back. Care should be taken that the arms are kept squarely against the ears. The motion should be like waving the mast of a ship, the hips representing the deck, while the trunk, head, and arms up to the top of the hands, represent the mast. This movement, like the others, should not be extreme at first, but gradually increased after a week or so.

Weave: (The order is "Weave. Ready - Cross. Weave!") Assume the "Cross" position. In this movement, at "Cross" the feet are spread until the heels are about twelve inches apart. The left foot remains stationary, the right foot being moved to accomplish this. On a count of "One, two, three, four" the body is turned to the left from the hips, the arms maintaining the same relation to the shoulders as at "Cross," until at "One" the face is to the left, the right arm pointing straight forward (in relation to the feet) and the left arm straight backward. (See Fig. 13.)

At "Two" the body is bent from the waist so that the right arm goes down and the left up; and at "Three" the fingers of the right hand touch the ground midway between the feet. The left arm should then be pointing straight up, with the face still to the left. The right knee must be slightly bent to accomplish this position. (See Fig. 14.)

In the "Weave" care should be taken that the arms and shoulders are kept in one line. The turn begins with the arms horizontal until they are nearly at right angles to the "Cross" position. Then the knee commences to bend and the body bends at the trunk, the hip turning in until the finger tips touch the floor. At that time the arms and shoulders should still be in the same relative position as at the start - namely, in "Cross" position.]

At "Four" the position of "Cross" is resumed, and on a count of "One, two, three, four" the same movement is repeated, this time with the left hand touching the ground. Throughout the exercise care should be taken that the arms remain in the same straight line, making no separate movement, but changing their position only as the trunk and shoulders are moved and carry the arms along. After this exercise has been thoroughly mastered, the turning and bending movements made on the counts "One" and "Two" should be combined - *i.e.*, instead of making the entire turn, as described above, turn and bend simultaneously. The entire movement should be repeated ten times.

In the "Weave" care should be taken that the arms and shoulders are kept in one line. The turn begins with the arms horizontal until they are nearly at right angles to the "Cross" position. Then the knee commences to flex and the body bends at the trunk, the hip turning in until the finger-tips touch the floor. At that time the arms and shoulders should still be in the same relative position as at the start - namely, in "Cross" position.

Wing: ( The order is  "Wing. Ready - Cross. Arms up.

Wing!") This is a finishing exercise consisting of deep breathing and is performed slowly. On a count of "One, two, three, four" the arms are raised laterally until they are extended straight upward at "One" and a full inhalation is reached. (See Fig. 15.) At "Two" the arms begin to fall forward and downward, and the body bends forward from the waist up, and eyes front, until, at "Four" the body has reached the limit of motion and the arms have passed the sides and have been forced back and up (as the trunk assumes a horizontal position) as far as possible. (See Fig. 15a.)

In the "Wing" position, which is a final breathing exercise, the breath should be taken well in as the arms are raised over the head; then exhaled as the body and arms swing forward, with a final crowding out of some of the residual air by forcing in the abdomen as the arms are raised over the back. Start the inhalation again as the arms come forward.]

On a count of "One, two, three, four" the body is straightened, reaching an upright position, with arms vertically extended, at "Three." At "Four" the arms are lowered to a "Cross" position, but with palms up and arms and shoulders forced hard back. Very slow counting is essential to the correct execution of this exercise. All air should be forced from the lungs as the body bends forward to the "Wing" position, and they should be filled to capacity as the body is straightened and the arms brought down. Inhale through the nose. The entire movement should be repeated five times.

## HEALTH MAXIMS

Preparedness    is    nine-tenths    physical    strength

and endurance.

If you take more food than the digestion can handle, you not only tire the stomach, but the whole system.

Envy, jealousy, and wrath will ruin any digestion.

You'll never get the gout from walking.

Tennis up to the thirties, but golf after forty.

Tight shoes have sent many a man to bed with a cold.

Leg weariness never yet produced brain fag.

Whenever you walk, stand up, with chin in, hips back, and chest out, and think how tall you are.

Courage and concentration will conquer most obstacles.

The hurry of half a squad never brought the whole troop home.

The army must have sound lungs and a good stomach quite as much as arms and ammunition.

# Choose from Thousands of 1stWorldLibrary Classics By

Adolphus WilliamWard
Aesop
Agatha Christie
Alexander Aaronsohn
Alexander Kielland
Alexandre Dumas
Alfred Gatty
Alfred Ollivant
Alice Duer Miller
Alice Turner Curtis
Alice Dunbar
Ambrose Bierce
Amelia E. Barr
Andrew Lang
Andrew McFarland Davis
Anna Sewell
Annie Besant
Annie Hamilton Donnell
Annie Payson Call
Anton Chekhov
Arnold Bennett
Arthur Conan Doyle
Arthur Ransome
Atticus
B. M. Bower
Basil King
Bayard Taylor
Ben Macomber
Booth Tarkington
Bram Stoker
C. Collodi
C. E. Orr
C. M. Ingleby
Carolyn Wells
Catherine Parr Traill
Charles A. Eastman
Charles Dickens
Charles Dudley Warner
Charles Farrar Browne
Charles Ives
Charles Kingsley
Charles Lathrop Pack
Charles Whibley
Charles Willing Beale
Charlotte M. Braeme
Charlotte M.Yonge
Clair W. Hayes
Clarence Day Jr.
Clarence E. Mulford

Clemence Housman
Confucius
Cornelis DeWitt Wilcox
Cyril Burleigh
D. H. Lawrence
Daniel Defoe
David Garnett
Don Carlos Janes
Donald Keyhole
Dorothy Kilner
Dougan Clark
E. Nesbit
E.P.Roe
E. Phillips Oppenheim
Edgar Allan Poe
Edgar Rice Burroughs
Edith Wharton
Edward J. O'Biren
John Cournos
Edwin L. Arnold
Eleanor Atkins
Elizabeth Cleghorn
Gaskell
Elizabeth Von Arnim
Ellem Key
Emily Dickinson
Erasmus W. Jones
Ernie Howard Pie
Ethel Turner
Ethel Watts Mumford
Eugenie Foa
Eugene Wood
Evelyn Everett-Green
Everard Cotes
F. J. Cross
Federick Austin Ogg
Ferdinand Ossendowski
Francis Bacon
Francis Darwin
Frances Hodgson Burnett
Frank Gee Patchin
Frank Harris
Frank Jewett Mather
Frank L. Packard
Frederick Trevor Hill
Frederick Winslow Taylor
Friedrich Kerst
Friedrich Nietzsche
Fyodor Dostoyevsky

Gabrielle E. Jackson
Garrett P. Serviss
Gaston Leroux
George Ade
Geroge Bernard Shaw
George Ebers
George Eliot
George MacDonald
George Orwell
George Tucker
George W. Cable
George Wharton James
Gertrude Atherton
Grace E. King
Grant Allen
Guillermo A. Sherwell
Gulielma Zollinger
Gustav Flaubert
H. A. Cody
H. B. Irving
H. G. Wells
H. H. Munro
H. Irving Hancock
H. Rider Haggard
H. W. C. Davis
Hamilton Wright Mabie
Hans Christian Andersen
Harold Avery
Harold McGrath
Harriet Beecher Stowe
Harry Houidini
Helent Hunt Jackson
Helen Nicolay
Hendy David Thoreau
Henrik Ibsen
Henry Adams
Henry Ford
Henry Frost
Henry James
Henry Jones Ford
Henry Seton Merriman
Henry Wadsworth
Longfellow
Henry W Longfellow
Herbert A. Giles
Herbert N. Casson
Herman Hesse
Homer
Honore De Balzac

Horace Walpole
Horatio Alger, Jr.
Howard Pyle
Howard R. Garis
Hugh Lofting
Hugh Walpole
Humphry Ward
Ian Maclaren
Israel Abrahams
J.G.Austin
J. Henri Fabre
J. M. Barrie
J. Macdonald Oxley
J. S. Knowles
J. Storer Clouston
Jack London
Jacob Abbott
James Allen
James Lane Allen
James Andrews
James Baldwin
James DeMille
James Joyce
James Oliver Curwood
James Oppenheim
James Otis
Jane Austen
Jens Peter Jacobsen
Jerome K. Jerome
John Burroughs
John F. Kennedy
John Gay
John Glasworthy
John Habberton
John Joy Bell
John Milton
John Philip Sousa
Jonathan Swift
Joseph Carey
Joseph Conrad
Joseph Jacobs
Julian Hawthrone
Julies Vernes
Justin Huntly McCarthy
Kakuzo Okakura
Kenneth Grahame
Kate Langley Bosher
L. A. Abbot
L. T. Meade
L. Frank Baum
Laura Lee Hope

Laurence Housman
Leo Tolstoy
Leonid Andreyev
Lewis Carroll
Lilian Bell
Lloyd Osbourne
Louis Tracy
Louisa May Alcott
Lucy Fitch Perkins
Lucy Maud Montgomery
Lydia Miller Middleton
Lyndon Orr
M. H. Adams
Margaret E. Sangster
Margaret Vandercook
Maria Edgeworth
Maria Thompson Daviess
Mariano Azuela
Marion Polk Angellotti
Mark Overton
Mark Twain
Mary Austin
Mary Cole
Mary Rowlandson
Mary Wollstonecraft
Shelley
Max Beerbohm
Myra Kelly
Nathaniel Hawthrone
O. F. Walton
Oscar Wilde
Owen Johnson
P.G.Wodehouse
Paul and Mable Thorn
Paul G. Tomlinson
Paul Severing
Peter B. Kyne
Plato
R. Derby Holmes
R. L. Stevenson
Rabindranath Tagore
Rahul Alvares
Ralph Waldo Emmerson
Rene Descartes
Rex E. Beach
Richard Harding Davis
Richard Jefferies
Robert Barr
Robert Frost
Robert Gordon Anderson
Robert L. Drake

Robert Lansing
Robert Michael Ballantyne
Robert W. Chambers
Rosa Nouchette Carey
Ross Kay
Rudyard Kipling
Samuel B. Allison
Samuel Hopkins Adams
Sarah Bernhardt
Selma Lagerlof
Sherwood Anderson
Sigmund Freud
Standish O'Grady
Stanley Weyman
Stella Benson
Stephen Crane
Stewart Edward White
Stijn Streuvels
Swami Abhedananda
Swami Parmananda
T. S. Ackland
The Princess Der Ling
Thomas A. Janvier
Thomas A Kempis
Thomas Anderton
Thomas Bailey Aldrich
Thomas Bulfinch
Thomas De Quincey
Thomas H. Huxley
Thomas Hardy
Thomas More
Thornton W. Burgess
U. S. Grant
Valentine Williams
Victor Appleton
Virginia Woolf
Walter Scott
Washington Irving
Wilbur Lawton
Wilkie Collins
Willa Cather
Willard F. Baker
William Makepeace
Thackeray
William W. Walter
Winston Churchill
Yei Theodora Ozaki
Young E. Allison
Zane Grey